Computers in Psychiatry

Computers in Psychiatry

Edited by Fionnbar Lenihan

Gaskell

Gaskell is an imprint of the Royal College of Psychiatrists, 17 Belgrave Square, London SW1X 8PG
http://www.rcpsych.ac.uk

British Library Cataloguing-in-Publication Data.
A catalogue record for this book is available from the British Library.
ISBN 1-904671-21-7

Distributed in North America by Balogh International Inc.

The views presented in this book do not necessarily reflect those of the Royal College of Psychiatrists, and the publishers are not responsible for any error of omission or fact.

The editor and authors have declared no pecuniary interests in any of the products discussed.

The Royal College of Psychiatrists is a registered charity (no. 228636).

This publication is dedicated to Marie.

Printed by Bell & Bain Limited, Glasgow, UK.

Contents

Contributors

Bettadapura Ashim, Specialist Registrar in General Adult & Forensic Psychiatry, Edenfield Centre, Prestwich Hospital, Manchester; ashim@nhs.net

Sindhu Ashim, Consultant Psychiatrist, The Spinney, Everest Road, Manchester; sindhu.ashim@nhs.net

John Bourke, Founder of Nichiai, a Tokyo-based marketing, IT services and consulting firm; johnb@nichiai.com

Conor Darcy, Chief Technical Officer, D'Arcy Software Group; conor.darcy@gmail.com

Martin Elphick, Consultant in General Adult Psychiatry and Chair of the Royal College of Psychiatrists Informatics Committee.

Matt Evans, Old Age Psychiatrist and former Chair of Mental Health Informatics Special Interest Group of the Royal College of Psychiatrists; matt.evans@nhs.net

Gurpal Singh Gosall, Consultant Psychiatrist, Queen's Park Hospital, Blackburn, Lancashire; gsg@gosall.com

David Harris, Barrister (specialising in IT, Internet and intellectual property law; psybook@ukitlaw.com

Stuart Leask, Senior Lecturer in Psychiatry, University of Nottingham; Honorary Consultant in Rehabilitation Psychiatry; stuart.leask@nottingham.ac.uk

Fionnbar Lenihan, Consultant Forensic Psychiatrist, The Orchard Clinic, Royal Edinburgh Hospital; fionnbar@cix.co.uk

Michael G. Madden, Lecturer in Information Technology, National University of Ireland, Galway, Ireland; michael.madden@nuigalway.ie

Justine McCulloch, Consultant Psychiatrist, NHS Forth Valley, Scotland; justine.mcculloch@nhs.net

Bruce Taylor, General Practitioner Trainee, Northumbria; Gaskell@BruceTaylor.co.uk

Karen Tingay, Technical Project Coordinator for the CAMHS Outcomes Research Consortium, University College London; rejukst@ucl.ac.uk

James Woolley, Clinical Research Fellow, Institute of Psychiatry and Specialist Registrar, Maudsley Hospital, London; j.woolley@iop.kcl.ac.uk

Preface

Fionnbar Lenihan

Why this book?

You have purchased, or are considering purchasing, this Gaskell book with the familiar College crest. Moreover, it's about, of all things, computers! Surely, an excessive interest in computers marks a person out as socially inept, incapable of normal human relationships, perhaps even suffering from some sort of empathy disorder. Why would a sensitive individual such as you risk such a fate?

It was to avoid such accusations that we made the focus of this book the psychiatry and not the computers. To this end we have been fortunate to receive contributions from doctors, lawyers and businesspersons as well as computer science professionals: contributions that do not idolise technology for its own sake but place it firmly in a social and organisational context.

In the following chapters you will read expert advice on how to select a computer for your home or office (Chapter 2), will be shown how to use common office applications to support your professional work (Chapters 3 to 6) and will learn how to use statistical and bibliographic tools (Chapters 7 and 8), to supplement your computer with a personal digital assistant (PDA) (Chapter 9) and use the World Wide Web and email effectively (Chapters 10 and 11).

While the shelves in bookshops groan under the weight of computer manuals and how-to books, this is the only book to address computers and information technology (IT) more widely in terms of the tasks that a busy psychiatrist might want to perform.

In addition to these tutorial chapters, we are fortunate to have chapters covering the complex area of IT law as it might apply to psychiatrists, the need for security and the managerial and organisational problems that IT deployment might pose to an organisation (Chapters 12 to 14).

The tectonic collision of demographic trends and increasing expectations is squeezing health budgets all over the developed world. Efficiency savings are needed and it is likely that the slimmed down, nimble health services of the future will need more, not less, IT (see Chapter 15). It is unlikely, therefore, given the pressures to deliver improved health services, that psychiatrists will be left alone in a sort of tweedy backwater of paper charts and handwritten correspondence forever. Far better then to jump rather than be pushed. You can at least choose where you land!

For whom is this book intended?

The authors and the editor have an obvious personal interest in this book being purchased by as wide an audience as possible. Nevertheless, there are degrees of suitability and, setting aside our own interests, we would see the main market for this book being psychiatrists and, to a slightly lesser extent, doctors in other specialties.

Modern computers and operating systems make it easy to get started with a computer but our experience in the Royal College of Psychiatrists' Computers in Psychiatry Special Interest Group (CIPSIG; now the Mental Health Informatics Special Interest Group (MHISIG)) over the years has been that many users end up on a 'competence plateau', where further progress is painfully slow. We believe that the key to boosting competence in this group of busy professionals is to provide concise, readable, task-specific information relevant to their professional lives.

In addition to existing College members it is anticipated that the book will be of interest to new members as they enter the higher training grades and encounter, for perhaps the first time, managerial, audit and research duties that require the use of computers.

Fellow mental health professionals in nursing, social work and psychology have IT needs that are very similar to those of psychiatrists and this book will, we hope, be of interest to them as well.

How to read this book

To get the most from this book, readers should be able to start their computer, connect to the internet or local area network, create and organise files and folders (directories), start applications (programs) and produce and save files using these programs.

For any readers who feel that they might be a little behind in any of these areas, Chapter 1 offers a quick refresher course in these basic skills. Those who feel confident in their abilities can skip ahead.

Commercial reality dictated that Microsoft Windows and Microsoft Office applications are the examples most often used throughout this book, although we took care to ensure that those using alternatives such as Macintosh computers or Linux were not excluded.

A recent trend has been the release of high-quality free or 'open source' software ('free' both in the monetary sense and in the sense of being free of restrictive licensing). We believe that this collaborative approach to software development has much to recommend it and we have highlighted where these options are available.

There is a logical progression to the chapters in this book, starting off with the basics of using a computer and moving on to buying a computer and then doing various useful things before, in the last few chapters, standing back and looking at the big picture. However, you may want just to dip into chapters that interest you and leave the rest for later.

Aims

Our goal in producing this book, is that you, the reader, will be empowered to accomplish one of your own goals. This goal might be as simple as creating a professional-looking curriculum vitae or as complex as doing multivariate analysis on a data-set.

When you've finished

Gaskell maintains a website for this book, which you can find (or will be able to find after you have read the book) at *http://www.rcpsych.ac.uk/computers_and_internet_psychiatry*. We have links to software mentioned in the book as well as templates and sample materials created by the authors.

There is also a discussion forum where you can discuss issues related to computers in psychiatry and post questions. We cannot guarantee support (we have day jobs!) but there's a good chance you will find the answer you're looking for.

If the book stimulates your interest in psychiatric computing, you might want to join the MHISIG. You are very welcome to join even if you are not a member of the Royal College of Psychiatrists (or even not a psychiatrist). You can find a link to the membership page at *http://www.rcpsych.ac.uk/college/sig/comp/*.

Finally, we have done our best to catch errors and typographical mistakes but we might have missed a few. Mail bug reports, praise, complaints and hate mail to fionnbar@cix.co.uk.

Acknowledgements

I gratefully acknowledge the support of the Aberdeen and Tayside Higher Professional Psychiatric Training Schemes in the production of this book. I particularly thank Dr John Boyd, Director of the Aberdeen Forensic Psychiatry Training Scheme, for his encouragement.

Computers in Psychiatry emerged from the matrix of the CIPSIG (now MHISIG) of the Royal College of Psychiatrists, although the actual idea of writing a book about computers for psychiatrists had its origins in a converstaion with Dr Sudhir Kaligotla (committee member of the then CIPSIG. Dr Kaligotla's contribution is gratefully acknowledged.

Finally, I thank my wife Marie for her patience during the prolonged gestation of this book.

Fionnbar Lenihan
December 2005

CHAPTER 1

Basics

Fionnbar Lenihan and Conor Darcy

Opening the box

You've just taken delivery of your first computer – congratulations! Whether a desktop or laptop, Windows or Mac, it may be a whole new world to you, with lots of disks and leaflets and puzzling bits to connect. So what have you got for your money?

The various pieces are illustrated in Fig. 1.1. The large squarish box houses the main processing unit and other components that make a computer work. It will also have lots of sockets of varying shapes and sizes on one or more sides. We'll call this box alone the 'computer' from now on.

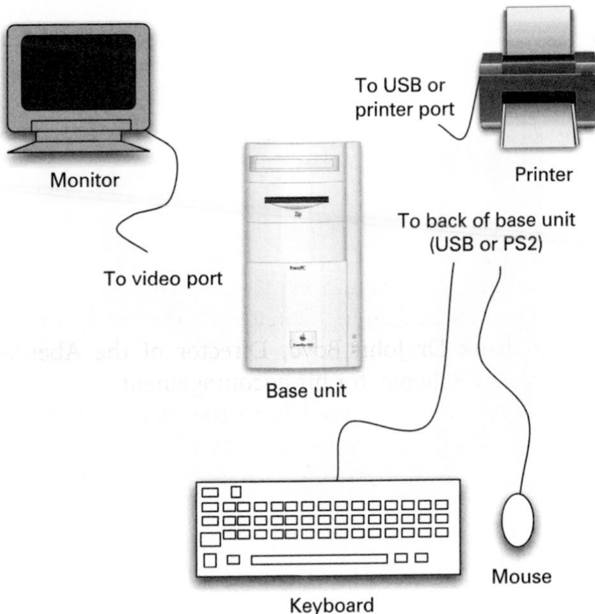

Fig. 1.1 The parts of a typical computer.

Connecting it all together

Some of the sockets and cables you see may already be familiar to you, for example if the power cable is not in-built it will have a socket similar to those found on kettles. Other than for power, the remaining sockets are for transferring information and are referred to as 'ports' in the world of information technology (IT) (Fig. 1.2). The good news is that these ports are designed to make it very hard for the wrong connectors to fit, so if something fits easily, it is probably in the right place.

Put the computer where you intend to use it. Leave enough room at the front for the keyboard and mouse, with the latter offset to the right or left depending on whether you are right- or left-handed.

One of your boxes will have contained a monitor (screen), either a large cathode ray tube (CRT) unit (like a traditional television) or a newer flat-screen unit. In either case, it should come with a cable with a connector at the end (one with pins sticking out of it) that looks suspiciously like it could be inserted into the monitor port. Note that the monitor port has holes for pins while the connector has the pins (Fig. 1.3). Place the monitor where you will be able to see it clearly without straining your neck. Connect it to the computer.

Now place the keyboard and mouse where you intend to use them. Most keyboards and mice have one cable each that cannot be disconnected, the other end of which terminates in either a roundish 'PS2' connector or a

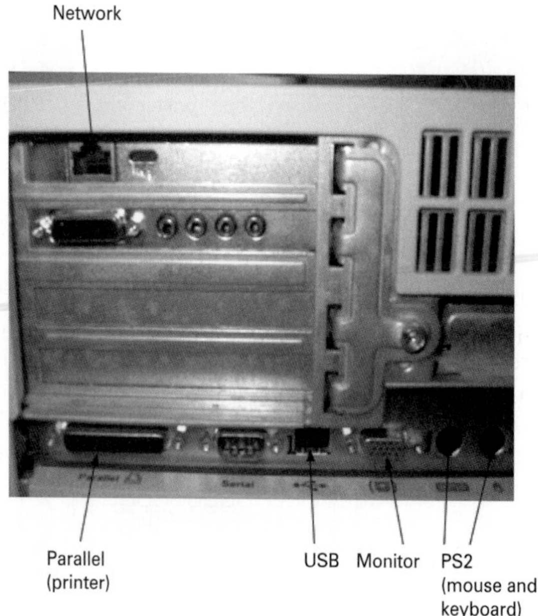

Fig. 1.2 Ports.

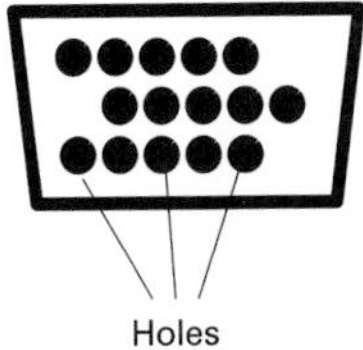

Fig. 1.3 Diagram of monitor port.

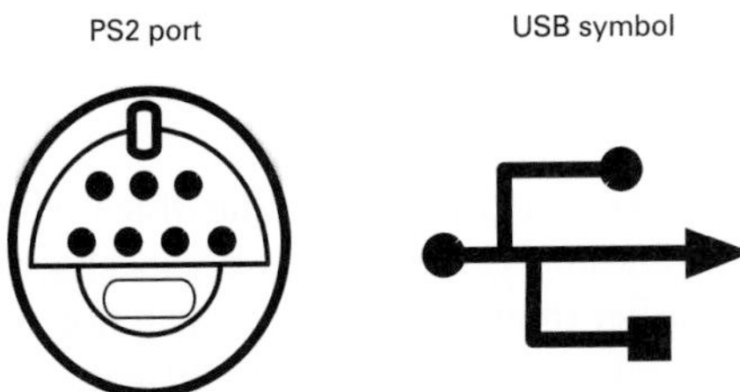

Fig. 1.4 Diagram of PS2 port and the USB symbol.

flat rectangular USB (universal serial bus) connector. Colour codes or little pictures are sometimes provided to show you what goes where. The USB ports and cables are also sometimes labelled with the rather arcane symbol shown in Fig. 1.4.

Similarly, if you have a printer or scanner, position it appropriately and hook it up (usually with a USB cable). It will likely need a power cable too.

Take some time to make sure that you will be comfortable with the layout of the components. If some of your ports are at the back of the computer, reposition the computer so that you have easy access.

If you have an in-built modem, your computer will have a port just like the standard analogue telephone jack in the wall. This varies from country to country. You can run a phone cable from the modem port to the phone socket on your wall. You will also need the settings your modem uses to communicate with your internet service provider (ISP). These details may be supplied in print form by your ISP or, more commonly these days, incorporated into an automated program that will do the configuration for you. In contrast a typical work set-up will involve a local area network (LAN) connection instead of a modem connection. For use in such a setting, your computer must have a LAN card, which you can determine by checking for a LAN or network port on your computer (see Fig. 1.2). A LAN port accepts a LAN cable connector. If you are planning to connect to a LAN you must use the LAN port and LAN cable rather than the telephone/modem equivalents, even though the two may look somewhat similar. Most modern offices have LAN ports, usually found close to power sockets in the wall and/or phone sockets. If you have a LAN cable, connect one end to the LAN

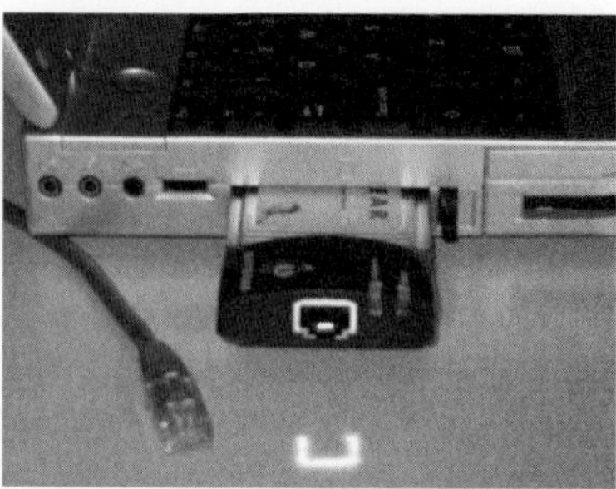

Fig. 1.5 PC network card and slot on a laptop computer.

port on your PC and the other to a LAN port in the office (check with your IT department that this is OK and get the necessary local settings).

If you bought a laptop rather than a desktop, you will not need a separate monitor, keyboard or mouse. However, for ergonomic reasons, many laptop users also use external versions of these. Thus a laptop is likely to have the same ports as those described for a desktop computer, but some of these will be on PC 'cards' instead of being built into the computer. A PC card is a way of providing extra functionality to a laptop. These flat, credit-card-like cards plug into slots on the side of the laptop; typically a laptop will have two, one stacked on top of the other. To use a PC card, simply push the card into a free slot before connecting the cables to the ports as before (Fig. 1.5).

The next step with either a laptop or a desktop computer is to check that all the peripheral devices are connected, including the monitor. Plug in all the relevant power cables and switch on the computer and other devices.

Welcome to the world of computing!

Other types of computer

Most people will be familiar with laptop and desktop computers as described above. You may also see 'tablet' PCs which are like A4 pads on which you write rather than type.

Starting up

When you turn on the power to a computer there is typically a delay of a minute or so before it becomes usable (while it 'boots up'). This is due to the computer needing to do various housekeeping tasks, to check that it is working properly, and so on.

Most modern computers can be used by several different people, each with their own programs, files and so on. To ensure that the correct settings are loaded you will be asked to identify yourself at the end of the boot-up period. This is called 'logging on' or 'logging in'. If your computer is

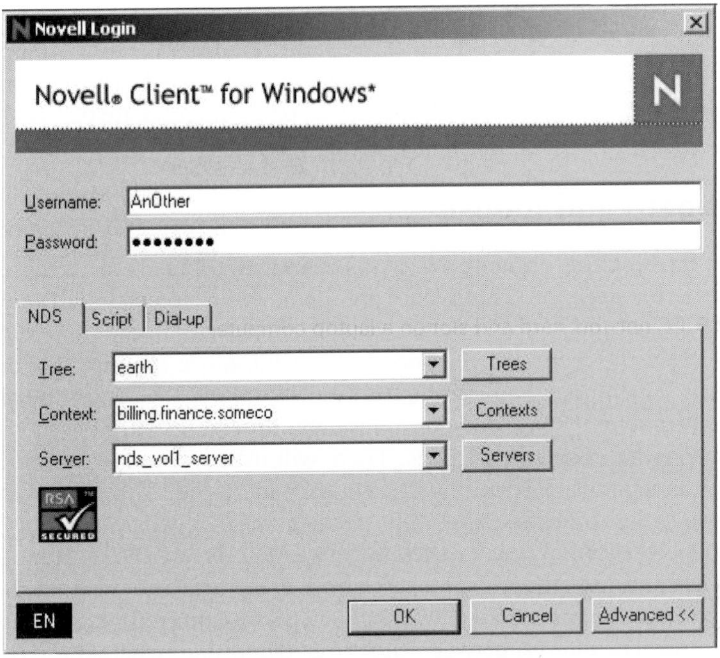

Fig. 1.6 Log-in screen.

connected to an office network this process can also be used to check that you are entitled to access the network.

Nowadays, most computers come with an operating system (the 'master program') pre-installed by the manufacturer. The first time the computer is powered up, it brings you through a series of steps designed to help you set up the computer the way you want it to be. The machine may have to be restarted (rebooted) during this process.

When a computer running the Windows XP operating system is started for the first time, you will be asked whether or not you wish to create a specially privileged user (the 'administrator') who can 'access all areas' and in general do anything. While this is necessary for maintenance and configuration it is a good idea (if slightly dissociative behaviour) also to create a second, 'ordinary' user account for regular day-to-day work, even if you are the only user of the machine, as this helps protect the computer against error and certain types of malice.

If you are logging into an office environment, you should already have been given a username, password and domain from your network administrator. If not, get this information from your administrator before you continue.

Make sure you are connected to the network (either with a LAN cable or wirelessly) and enter the username and password you were given. Once you have entered your username and password (see Fig. 1.6) you may be asked to change the password immediately. If so, you should either commit the new password to memory or record it in a secure location, as losing it may involve a time-consuming chase to find a person who can assign a new one! (See Mike Madden's guidance in Chapter 13 on creating secure passwords.)

Keyboard and mouse

At its simplest, pressing a key on the keyboard causes the corresponding letter to appear on the screen. Later on in this chapter we will show some simple editing to illustrate this (see 'Working with programs', below).

Hold the mouse in your dominant hand. Move the mouse around the mat. Watch how the mouse cursor moves around the screen in parallel. If you run out of space on your mouse mat lift and recentre the mouse upon it. Practise clicking on things. There will usually be at least two buttons (although most Mac mice will have only one). The left button is the main one. Unless otherwise specified, 'clicking' means clicking with this button. 'Double clicking' means clicking twice quickly on this button. Practise double clicking too; this is a sort of rapid 'tap-tap' movement of the finger and is quite a tricky manoeuvre, so don't get discouraged if it takes a while to master. The interval between clicks that determines whether the computer accepts two clicks as a double click or as two single clicks can vary (and can be altered). So, early on, you may think that you have double clicked to open an application, only to find that the computer is inviting you to rename something! Renaming is normally the result of two single clicks.

Now, time for a brief digression into philosophy, history and literary criticism!

The desktop and menu bar

Leaving aside difficult questions as to what, 'really', is reality, we can assert that what computers do, in reality, is arithmetic: counting on fingers – two fingers in fact. What makes computers useful is that they can do this really, really quickly. This binary finger counting is terribly dull, so much so that professional programmers have long since separated themselves from it by layers of translation. Programmers typically write software in vaguely English-like text. This is then converted, by special programs, into 0s and 1s that can be interpreted by the computer.

In the 1980s, when computers were being introduced to a sceptical public, it seemed natural to extend this process of abstraction, of metaphor creation, by further insulating the user from the reality of the machine. Thus was invented the graphical user interface (GUI). The most popular analogy was that of the 'desktop'. This (rather garbled) metaphor has the flat surface of the computer screen pretending to be an idealised desktop with various 'icons' (little pictures) representing objects on your computer or actions you

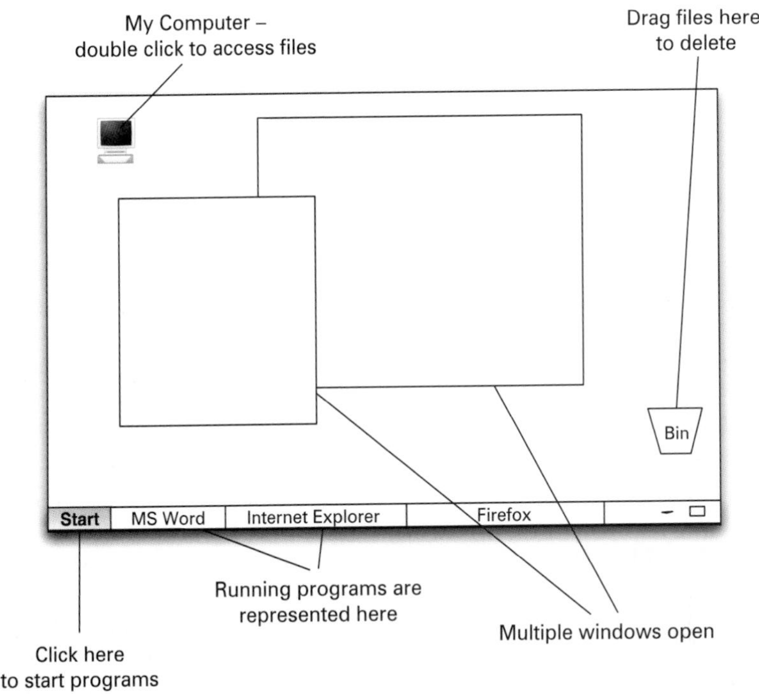

Fig. 1.7 A typical computer desktop.

can perform with those objects (we said it was a mixed metaphor). Clicking once on the relevant icon selects it; double clicking opens or activates it. When this happens a 'window' generally springs open that displays the contents of the object you opened or the action that you requested. Many windows can be open at once. Windows can overlap one another and can be 'minimised' or shrunk on to the little bar at the bottom of your screen.

Figure 1.7 shows a typical Windows desktop, but Macintosh, UNIX and other operating systems differ only in detail. Generally, a computer desktop will contain a way of accessing the file system (see below), a way of launching programs, a way of seeing what programs are currently running and miscellaneous things like a recycle bin.

Menus

Another more or less universal feature of a GUI is the so-called drop-down menu. This is illustrated in Fig. 1.8.

Click once on the menu title and the whole menu 'drops down' and further options can then be selected by further single clicks. Menus tend to be fairly consistent between programs, so that **Print** will almost always be

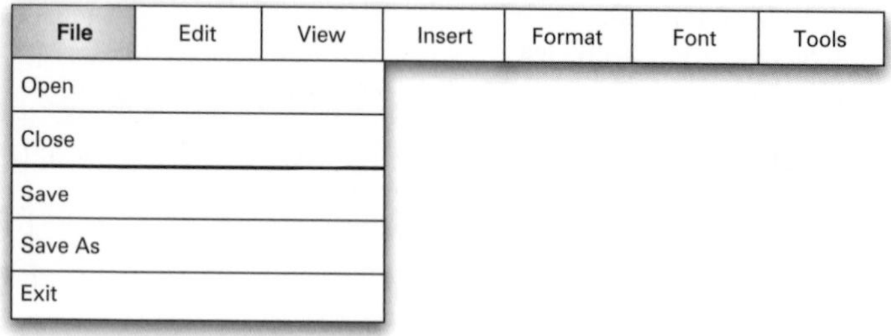

Fig. 1.8 A simple drop-down menu.

found under **File**. On computers running Windows, the drop-down menu will always be found at the top of the window you are using. On Macintosh computers, it will be found at the top of the screen as a whole.

Files and the file system

A file is a collection of related data, which are stored together, manipulated as a unit and given a single, unique, name. Generally a single file will contain a single document, so that *my_great_novel.doc* and *my_parlous_finances.xls* correspond to a masterpiece and a budget, respectively.

There are many types of file, which in GUIs are represented by different icons. This helps the user understand what type of file he or she is dealing with. Usually the icon corresponds to that of the program that can open the file. Another clue to a file's nature is the three-letter extension on the end. For example, a file ending *.exe* will be an 'executable' file – that is, a program. The most common file types are given in Table 1.1.

Folders (directories)

A directory or folder is just another file and it can be copied, moved and deleted in the usual way. Folders, however, have the special property of being able to contain other files 'inside' them, including other folders, which in turn can contain other folders, and so on (Fig. 1.9). Creating folders and sub-folders for the data files you create is a good idea because, just like a real filing system, it helps you keep track of things. Folders are represented both in Windows and on a Mac by a folder icon.

This folder-inside-folder arrangement creates a hierarchy (a concept familiar to those who work for the National Health Service!), which can be navigated in various ways.

On a Windows computer you can access the file system hierarchy by double clicking on the icon on your desktop labelled **My Computer**. A window will open, revealing an icon called either **Hard Drive** or **Main (C:)**. Open this in the same way. (On a Mac a similar action on the icon marked

Table 1.1 Common file types

Extension	File type/use	Programs to open	Comments
.jpeg, .jpg	Photographic images	Paintshop Pro, Photoshop	Your digital camera uses this
.gif	Non-photographic images (e.g. logos)	Paintshop Pro, Photoshop	
.doc	MS Word Documents	MS Word	Can also be opened by most other word processing programs
.rtf	Rich text file. Used as an exchange format for word processors	All word processors	Preserves some formatting
.txt	ASCII (plain text). Machine-readable files, 'lowest common denominator' exchange	All word processors, text editors	Preserves *no* formatting
.html, .htm	Web pages are written in this	Web browser	Basically text with funny tags
.xls	MS Excel spreadsheet	Excel	Can also be opened by OpenOffice
.ppt, .pps	MS PowerPoint	PowerPoint, other presentation software	.ppt is an editable presentation, .pps is a ready-to-go slide show
.pdf	Acrobat files. Used to circulate/ exchange documents where the formatting and appearance are not to change	Acrobat Reader	Also called 'Adobe' files
.mpg, .mpeg	International video standard	Real Player, Windows Media Player	
.mp3	Compressed music file	Real Player, Windows Media Player, iTunes	
.avi	Compressed movie file	Real Player, Windows Media Player	

Hard Drive will do the trick.) You will be rewarded with a vista of files and folders, most of which you will not recognise. These are mostly files used by the computer itself. It is OK to look at these but not a good idea to copy, move or delete them. You can, however, experiment in the folder marked **My Documents**.

You can open or enter folders by double clicking on their icons. If you find the window is too cramped, you can make it take up the whole screen by clicking on the icon that looks like a rectangle in the top-right corner of the

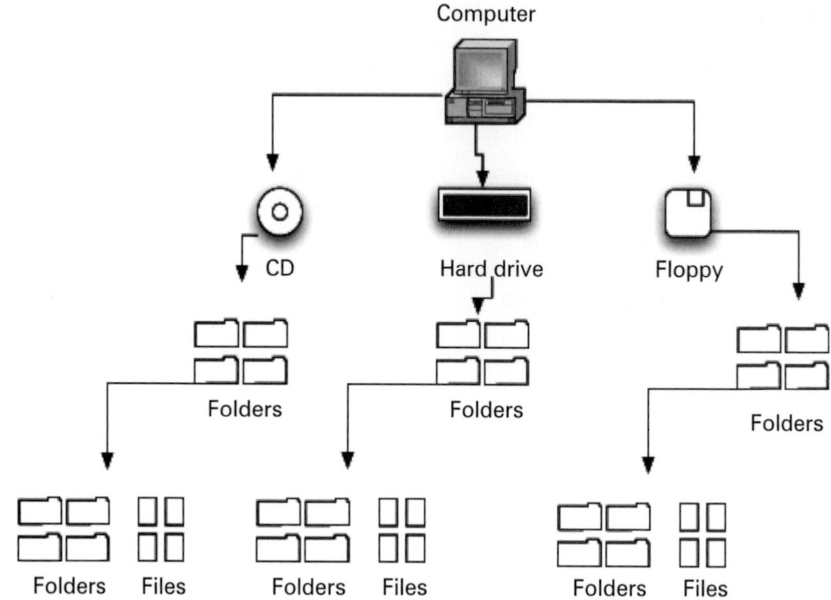

Fig. 1.9 The file system.

window. On a Mac this 'maximisation' of a window is accomplished with a single click on the + sign, which is the right-most of the three symbols at the top-left corner of the window.

To go 'up' the hierarchy (towards the root) in Windows you click on the icon marked 'up' in the middle of the bar along the top of the window. Finally, you can close the current window by single clicking on the box marked '×' in the top-right corner of the window. On a Mac there is no 'up' button as such, but you can jump all the way to the top by single clicking on the 'hard drive' icon, which can be found at the side of the window. If your Mac has a name this icon will be labelled with it. Alternatively, you can step 'up' the filesystem by pressing [Apple]+[pg up].

Creating folders

To create a new sub-folder within *My Documents* select **File → New → Folder** from the menu. The new folder will pop into existence but the name will be highlighted in blue, with a default of *New Folder*. Type a name in here and you're done. Go and make another folder. You're not likely to run out of room!

On a Mac you simply click on the title underneath the icon for the file you want to rename. It takes a little practice because it is all too easy to click on the icon itself, which is not what we want. If you click just right the title becomes highlighted, letting you type a new one.

Deleting files and folders

On a PC, to delete a file or folder you must indicate to the computer what file or folder it is you want to delete. You accomplish this selection process by single clicking with the left mouse button on the file in question. A blue box will surround it, indicating that the computer knows that you have selected it. Now select **File → Delete**. You will be asked if you are sure (a safety precaution), so click on the button marked *Yes*. That's it.

The Mac method is pretty much the same except that delete is referred to as **File → Move To Trash**.

Renaming files

Follow the procedure for deleting but choose **Rename** instead of **Delete** from the menu. The name will now be highlighted in blue, awaiting your new name (much as for folder creation above).

Moving and copying files

Files can be moved and copied using a variety of methods, such as dragging and dropping. This, however, can give inconsistent results. One method that is more predictable is simply to highlight the file as above and select **Edit → Copy** or **Edit → Cut** (the latter method deletes the original) from the menu. Navigate to the destination folder and select **Edit → Paste**. This works both in Windows and on a Mac, although there is no **Cut** option on the Mac (just manually delete the original afterwards).

As you become more proficient, you may notice that there are some short pieces of text beside some menu choices, e.g. [CTRL] + [C] (or [Apple] + [C] on the Mac) beside **Edit → Copy**. This means that by holding down the [CTRL] key and then typing [C] you copy the selected text, without needing the mouse at all. The equivalent for pasting is [CTRL] + [V].

Multiple files

If you have many files to work with, you can speed things up by selecting multiple files to work on. To do this hold down the [CTRL] key (the [APPLE] key on a Mac) on your keyboard and click on the first file you want to work on, then the second and so on. Each file will become outlined in blue, indicating it has been selected. When you have all the files selected you can proceed just as for a single file. To deselect a file you have accidentally selected, simply click it again.

To copy a set of contiguous files or folders in a list, hold down the [SHIFT] key and click on the first one you wish to copy and then on the last. All the others between will be selected too.

Removable storage

The most familiar form of removable storage is the humble floppy disk. Other types include CD–ROM, Zip drives, the little flash memory pen drives and memory cards (also commonly used in digital cameras).

Put the disk in the appropriate slot of your computer. Open **My Computer** as described above. You will see an icon representing the new disk. You can open this with the usual double click and do any of the file operations discussed above. In the case of CDs you cannot copy or move files to the CD or delete files from it since the CD is a form of 'read only memory' (ROM). (For simplicity we will ignore recordable CDs here.)

One of the most useful things you can do with removable storage is to make a copy of your most important files to protect against the loss or theft of your computer (a 'backup'). Mike Madden covers this in more detail in Chapter 13.

Applications (programs)

An application is another name for a program, such as your word processor or spreadsheet. Your PC will come preloaded with many applications. New applications can be downloaded from the internet or bought on CD from a shop.

Working with programs

On a Windows computer you can start most programs by clicking on the **Start** menu and selecting from the sub-menus thus revealed. The equivalent action on a Mac is to open the **Applications** folder.

Now start the Wordpad application. If you are using a Mac, start TextEdit. Spend a little time typing into the empty file that appears. Practise changing the appearance of the text using options from the drop-down menus. Now choose **Save As…** from the **File** menu. You will be asked to fill in boxes giving your newly created file a name and a location in the file system. Do remember what folder you put it in!

Now close the file by selecting **File** → **Close**. Open it again by choosing **File** → **Open**. Did you remember where you saved it?

Do a little more writing and choose **File** → **Save** from the menu. You will not be prompted for a name this time as the computer assumes you want to save to the current file.

It is important to realise that 'saving' in computer-speak is equivalent to erasing the original file and replacing it with the modified version. Therefore it can sometimes be sensible, when making a large change that you might regret later, to use **Save As…** to give the revised file a new name, so that you can revert to the original if needed.

For important documents it can also be useful sometimes to choose **Save As...** and save the file to an entirely different storage medium (e.g. to a network drive or to a floppy disk, if you are working normally on your own hard drive). This ensures that you will have a reasonably up-to-date file available, even if the main file becomes corrupted (unusable) because your storage medium fails. Many of us take this to heart only after having experienced such a failure at first hand, with the consequent loss of many hours' work.

Bear in mind also that in any particular folder there cannot be two files with the same name. Your computer will complain if you try to violate this rule. You may even succeed in erasing the contents of a file by writing another file over it.

When you are finished, leave the program by choosing **File** → **Exit** or **Application** → **Quit Application** on the Mac (where the **Application** is, say, Word).

Installing programs (applications)

The simplest kind of application consists of a single executable file, which you can run by double clicking on the appropriate icon, as discussed above. However, most applications are more complex than this, consisting of this core file and a host of supporting files (although you launch the program in the same way).

Putting all these files in the right place in the file system is a complex task that has long been automated. Most applications come packaged in a compressed form, usually with the extension *.zip* (on Windows or *.sit* or *.dmg* on Macs, or *.jar* for Java). This is uncompressed into a temporary folder using either the tools built into your computer or a program such as 7-Zip (*www.7-zip.org*). There may be a file called *readme.txt* that you should read (this computer stuff is hard!). You then usually double click on a special executable file in the resulting folder (usually called *Install.Exe* or *Setup.Exe*). This little program asks you a few questions (accepting the defaults is usually OK), puts all the files in the right place and creates an entry in the **Start** menu (bottom left of your screen) for Windows or in the **Applications** folder on a Mac. From here the new application can be conveniently started.

An alternative you sometimes see is the so-called 'self-extracting executable' file, where you simply double click on an executable file and it goes ahead and extracts and installs itself with no further need for you to do anything.

Installing programs is seductively easy. Removing them can be fiendishly difficult. Exercise restraint about what you install, particularly if you downloaded it from the internet. This is especially true for work machines, where you should get the permission of the IT staff before installing new software.

Network access

In an office environment the responsibility for maintaining network connections largely belongs to the professional administrators in the IT department. Once you have logged in (see above) you should be able to access any resources you are entitled to access, either on the local network or on the wider internet.

At home you will need to be your own network administrator. First, make sure you are physically connected to the internet, either by means of a telephone cable and modem or via a broadband (ADSL) modem. Insert the CD that was supplied by your ISP or that came with your modem (see above). It may then automatically open or you may have to open it from **My Computer → CD ROM**. The configuration program will be called *install* or *setup*. Run this by double clicking on it. If you run into problems there will usually be a helpline number on the CD or packaging.

Once the configuration program has finished, you will usually be able to activate the connection by clicking **My Computer → Dial Up Networking** and selecting it. Most programs that need an internet connection will start the connection themselves in any case.

To test your connection start Internet Explorer or another browser (see Chapter 10). If you have a valid connection you will see the text of the home page displayed. Links to other pages will be underlined in the text and displayed in a different colour. A single click on a link will cause that linked page to be loaded, replacing the current page.

Links need not only be to web pages. Photographs, videos, music and other files can also be stored on web servers (a server is a kind of 'workhorse' computer that 'serves' ordinary computers over a network) and linked to in the same manner. If the file type is one that the browser 'knows' how to handle, it will be displayed in the browser; otherwise a helper program will be launched or the file will simply be 'downloaded', that is, copied to your own computer. This, incidentally, is how programs and other files are obtained from the internet.

Sometimes you may wish to download a file straight away rather than have the browser try to open it. To ensure this occurs, click on the link using the right mouse button ([CTRL]+[CLICK] on a Mac). A menu will appear giving the option of saving the file.

It is important to try to remember in which folder the downloaded file was stored.

Miscellaneous terms

Those who work in IT are often accused of using an impenetrable jargon to mystify the public and enhance their own power and status. While such criticisms from sociologists, literary critics or even doctors invite a response incorporating the words 'kettle and 'pot', there are a couple of technical terms whose mastery will ease your entry into the world of IT.

The actual work of computing is done by a processor or 'chip'. Microscopic structures on the processor perform arithmetic using binary digits or bits (ones and zeroes). Eight of these bits make up a byte; 1 048 576 bytes make up a megabyte (MB) and 1024 million bytes comprise a gigabyte (GB).

The speed of a processor is measured in hertz with processors (at the time of writing) running at about 3–4 gigahertz (giga being the prefix for one billion).

Conclusion

This chapter covers a lot of ground, so don't be discouraged if you need to read it a couple of times. The effort will be worth it since once you have mastered these, basic, topics you will be well positioned to move on to the more interesting material in the remainder of the book.

CHAPTER 2

Buying a computer

John Bourke

Five or ten years ago, when personal computing had still not fully matured, choosing the right computer was a difficult task. However, since then computers have become commodities, and this has made it much easier to select a machine. Now almost every computer is capable of carrying out the majority of tasks for which people may wish to use it. Workstation functionality is effectively the same from maker to maker, with only differences in speed or storage space lending desktop computers any significant differentiation. The same applies to notebook computers, although with the additional dimension of weight becoming a factor. So, it is only for server and tablet PCs that there is much difference between makes and models. (See Chapter 1 for definitions of these different kinds of computer.)

For most people considering a purchase, this leaves only one barrier: the 'if I wait a little longer won't I be able to get a better machine?' feeling. Technology continues to evolve at the same pace it always has since computers came on to the market. However, if you want to buy a computer, it is important not to wait for new technologies to arrive, since technologies are always improving and the wait will never end. That said, currently the application of technological advances is, essentially, limited to performance enhancements and there are few new technologies leading to increased functionality. This, coupled with the fact that most improvements are only incremental, makes buying now as good a time as any. Prices are also not likely to drop significantly as margins are small and although the semi-conductor industry is somewhat cyclical (with, traditionally, a 4-year period with peaks coinciding with the Olympic Games), recent over-capacity has kept prices near rock-bottom levels.

For those of us who think performance is getting better and it might be prudent to wait a little longer, we need only to reflect on what is known as 'Moore's law'. In 1965 Gordon Moore, co-founder of Intel, observed that the number of transistors that could be squeezed on to a chip was doubling every couple of years and predicted that this trend would continue. 'Moore's law', as it was dubbed by the press, still holds true today and will probably not be invalidated in this decade. If, in the 1980s, people decided to postpone the purchase of a new computer until the 'next major breakthrough' was made, they would still be waiting today!

In summary, if you need a computer, buy one. It is not worth the wait.

Technical stuff

For those who wish to know a little more about what they are buying, there are three main components to be concerned with: memory, hard disk and processor.

Memory

As a former designer of computer memory, I feel well qualified to state that there is little a buyer needs to know about memory other than 'the more the better'. There are different types of memory and memories that have different speeds, but all that somebody buying a computer needs to know is that the more memory a computer has, the faster it can operate and the more complex are the tasks it can handle. For people wishing to do graphically intensive work – for example image analysis or playing games – the same rule applies for memory that is dedicated to handling the information that is used to display images on the screen (known as 'graphics memory' or 'video memory'). Video control systems that are integrated into the motherboard (the main circuit board to which other devices are connected) may be sufficient for some uses, and laptops tend to have everything on the motherboard. However, few workstations come with integrated video nowadays.

Hard disks

Hard disks (or 'hard drives') are somewhat more complex than memory. In addition to needing to worry about how much storage space they have (again, the more the better), there is also the question of speed. The speed at which the disk rotates (given in rpm) influences how fast data can be written and read. Here the rule, not surprisingly, is 'the faster the better'. If you plan on editing movies regularly on your computer, you will need a hard drive that is both as fast and as large as you can afford or have more than one. However, for most applications the differences will not be noticeable.

Processors

The processor is by far the most complex of the three components with which we are concerned. On the market there are processors from different makers, processors that have different architectures, different speeds and even ones that use what could be called different philosophies!

In broad terms, processors can be classified into two families; CISC (complex instruction set computing) processors and RISC (reduced instruction set computing) processors. Processors from Intel and from AMD are the former, while Motorola and IBM make processors that are the latter. The differences, although interesting, are beyond the scope of this chapter and for the vast majority of people there is no need even to be aware of the difference – the terms are mentioned here only for completeness and to help give confidence to anyone who may come across them elsewhere. However, having mentioned them, we may as well note that Macintosh computers use RISC processors and PCs use CISC processors (although at the time of writing Apple announced that future Macintosh computers would also use Intel CISC processors).

What we need to know to evaluate a processor is the amount of information it can process 'in one go', the length of time each 'go' takes, and the amount of cache (memory that is built into the processor that is used as a kind of notepad by the 'processing' part of the processor) it has. Let's get familiar with these in reverse order.

Processors have cache memory built in since write and read times to it are much faster than those to and from main memory. There are various degrees of proximity to the registers (the places where calculations are performed) and so there are different levels of cache, known with great imagination as 'level 1', 'level 2' and 'level 3', or L1, L2 and L3. As with main memory, the more cache memory the better. However, cache sizes will be reflected in the price of the processor.

The amount of time it takes a processor to complete an operation is determined by the speed of its internal clock. Each register can be used once per clock cycle or 'tick' as it were. The faster the clock ticks, the faster work is performed. Processor speeds have increased from about 33 MHz (megahertz, or million cycles per second) to 3.4 GHz (gigahertz, or thousand million cycles per second) in the past ten years. This means the clocks are ticking very quickly indeed. Although these numbers cease to have meaning to most of our minds, we need only remember the faster the better.

The last processor feature we need to consider is its architecture – how many bits of information it can process in one go. As a rule, all processors on the market are the same in this respect. However, there are occasional 'jumps' when the industry moves to a larger data 'mouthful'. At the time of writing, we are at the beginning of such a transition, with a move from a 32- to a 64-bit architecture, doubling the size of the mouthful. While 64-bit processors have an advantage over 32-bit ones, it is not a simple 'times two' advantage since, if the data being manipulated are less than 32 bits, a 64-bit processor is no faster than one taking 32-bit 'mouthfuls'. However, 64-bit processors have a major advantage in that they can address more memory, reducing the need to use the hard disk as temporary storage (known as 'virtual memory') if working with more than 4 gigabytes (GB) of data. As virtual memory is about 40 times slower than real memory, this is a considerable advantage for people who need high-end performance. At the time of writing, the main application of 64-bit processing is for servers, not workstations, though this will change.

Summary

To summarise all this technical information simply: we need to remember that we should get as much memory and hard disk storage capacity as our budget permits, that a hard disk that spins faster has an advantage over one that spins slower, and that processors – within the same architecture (32 bit or 64 bit) – with a faster clock speed and more cache are superior to ones with slower speeds and less cache.

Finally, there is one more impact that processor architecture has on our computing – software compatibility. AMD and Intel now both have 64-bit processors that are backward compatible with 32-bit software. However, 32-bit software running on a 64-bit platform cannot harness the full potential of 64-bit computing. At time of writing, Macintosh and Microsoft have both released 64-bit operating systems (Mac OS X Panther, MAC OS X, Windows Server 2003 and the 64-bit version of Windows XP), all of which support 32- and 64-bit software applications, there are 64-bit versions of the LINUX operating system and the upcoming Windows Vista is 64 bit. However, 64-bit software applications – of which very few currently exist – will not be backward compatible, that is to say they will not work on 32-bit computers.

There are many other technical details which are important, such as the system bus (the internal information highway), the graphics card, and the ability to attach peripheral devices, but these vary little between the computers on sale at any particular time. This means that we are now ready to move on and find out how to select the computer for our needs.

Selecting your tribe

Although this may strike some as an odd heading, it is a reasonably accurate label for the first choice we need to make. The personal computer, the mouse, the concept of a graphical user interface with windows and many other innovations were brought into existence by the tribe of Steve Jobs and Apple. Had the company's strategy been different in the early 1980s, maybe we wouldn't have tribes to choose between, but Apple decided to keep its systems proprietary and by doing so enabled the rise of what was at first known as the IBM PC tribe, which mutated into the 'Wintel tribe' (from Windows and Intel) and is now simply the PC tribe, since AMD has managed to win a place at the table with Intel.

Selecting which tribe to pledge your allegiance to comes down to a matter of personal taste. The PC tribe is by far the larger; its members are less fanatical about their allegiance but tend to benefit from greater hardware flexibility, greater availability of software, and a greater ability to share documents, as most people use PCs. However, Apple offers some great products and people who use them love them.

If you have no overwhelming desire to belong to the Apple tribe, I would recommend joining the PC tribe, as it is easier (and cheaper) to find people who can troubleshoot problems with PCs and there is a greater variety of compatible hardware and software.

Selecting a desktop

Although frequently called 'desktops', the modern personal computer often sits on the floor, so I prefer the term 'workstation', which once upon a time was used to refer to high-end desktops used for engineering tasks. Selecting one does depend on its intended use. However, for most tasks – such as word processing, email and spreadsheets – any workstation will suffice. Consequently, a good rule of thumb for most people is not to buy at the leading edge but two or three steps down from it. This will give performance that is still robust enough to handle any software that comes to market in first few years after purchase, while not commanding the price premium of the very latest models. Only if you intend to use the workstation to carry out multiple number-crunching tasks simultaneously should you consider being closer to the leading edge. This paragraph is probably the single most important one for readers of this chapter who are planning to buy a computer. To reiterate – the best price–performance position with adequate 'future-proofing' is a couple of steps back from the leading edge.

Don't select a processor with the smallest amount of cache, and make sure that there is a sizeable hard disk and as much memory as you are prepared to pay for – and you have 'your machine'. If you wish to use it for photographs, video and scanning it is worthwhile ensuring that it has 'Firewire' capabilities. ('Firewire', or 'IE1394', is a fast data communication method.)

The only other consideration requiring some thought is the monitor. Cathode ray tube (CRT) monitors have traditionally been superior to liquid crystal display (LCD) ones, as they offer greater brightness, contrast and flexible resolutions. However, LCD monitors are now almost as good as CRTs and the best of them are no longer set at a fixed resolution. This means that there is only one trade-off to consider – price versus desk space. LCD monitors take up much less desk space but are more expensive. Regardless of whether you select a CRT or LCD monitor, you should try to get one as large as possible in terms of viewable area for your budget. This is measured by taking the diagonal distance from the bottom left to the top right of the screen's viewable area (in the same way as for a television screen). A 17-inch screen is fine for most people. Smaller screens should be avoided but larger ones can be useful for people doing scientific work, editing graphics or simply needing to look at a couple of things side by side (note that in extreme cases two monitors can be hooked up to a single computer and used simultaneously, but this normally requires a special graphics card).

Selecting a notebook computer

Unlike with workstations, there is no issue with selecting a monitor for notebooks (a term that has replaced 'laptops', as it is supposed to conjure up the image of a lighter laptop), since notebooks have an LCD monitor built in and since one LCD technology dominates the market. Notebook computers follow the same rules of thumb as workstations, but with the additional consideration of the trade-off between weight and screen size and built-in devices. Smaller notebooks can be very portable but may not have a floppy or CD drive built in. While this is convenient for some, for those who may wish to install software or exchange files other than by email it means adding in hardware and cables.

The final consideration is battery life, but it is always possible to have a second battery, so this is not the most important factor.

Selecting a tablet PC

Of all the computers available, the tablet PC is the only type that is not yet a true commodity. Tablet PCs, the latest addition to the mobile computing world, are mobile computers that have screens on which you can write. Extreme portability and the ability to use a stylus for input have resulted in tablet PCs attracting considerable interest in the healthcare sector. To select one, the first question we need to answer is whether we are happy to accept a slower processor, smaller screen, limited hard disk space and a higher price in exchange for an ultra-mobile computer that can take handwritten input. If not, then our decision is made – we need to buy a notebook.

For those who can live with this trade-off, we are in the market for a tablet PC. However, we need to be more careful in selecting our computer than when choosing a workstation or notebook as tablets are relatively new and there is still quite a lot of difference between models. This makes simple price comparisons difficult, as more often than not they will be 'apple and oranges' comparisons. Tablets are also the only kind of computer that it really is best to examine physically before purchase, and to test a few to get a good feeling for their comparative usability.

The first step in selecting a tablet PC is to decide whether we want a true tablet (known as a 'slate') or a convertible notebook-to-tablet. Slates are designed for maximum mobility and stylus input. If you want to use a mouse, keyboard or external monitor with a slate, you need to buy a 'docking station', which enables these devices to be attached. 'Convertibles' are ultra-light notebook computers that have a screen that can be manipulated to fold flat against the keyboard, providing a tablet-like system. If you need a keyboard available for use at a moment's notice, then a convertible is the way to go. However, if you plan to use the computer mainly while standing, for example while on a ward, then a slate might be the better option.

The second step is to determine weight and screen size. These are related. The screen needs to be large enough to use easily but small enough for the whole device to remain portable. Checking out a few computers should help you make this decision. Once you have selected the screen size, brightness is the next priority. Brighter screens are easier to work with, but brightness has an impact on battery life.

The next critical factor is the stylus. Before buying a tablet PC you should write a paragraph or two with the stylus to ensure that it feels comfortable enough to use for a couple hours and that it is easy to write with.

The penultimate checkpoint is durability. Slates tend to be more durable than convertibles and tablets with metal casings, not surprisingly, are more resistant to abuse than those with plastic casings. In addition, the hard disk should be 'shock mounted' as this greatly reduces the risk of disk failure if the computer gets a bang or is dropped. For convertibles, it is also wise to check what the life expectancy of the hinge is, that is, how many times the screen can be opened, twisted, locked into tablet mode and closed again. This should be at least 30 000 times. This will provide a minimum of 3 years of computing, 5 days a week, with 40 opening and closings per day (much heavier use than the average tablet will get).

Finally, consider what accessories are available for use with the machine.

In conclusion

If you follow the above guidelines you should have a workstation, notebook or tablet computer that will serve you well for the next few years and that will let you perform any of the tasks described in the remainder of this book.

CHAPTER 3

Word processing: the next steps

Fionnbar Lenihan

Why should you use a word processor?

Doctors are highly skilled (and usually highly paid) professionals. Basic economics would suggest that the doctor would be best employed doctoring while someone else is paid to do the typing. In some circumstances, however, this simplistic analysis falls down.

Many psychiatrists do a small amount of private practice, perhaps in the form of medico-legal work. Unless you do a lot, however, it probably won't be worthwhile employing a secretary. Similar considerations apply to academic work, such as research or audit, where there may be limited or no secretarial support.

Unless you have an immense working memory, it is hard to keep the whole of a complex document in mind at once. A Dictaphone is inherently linear, while your thinking may not be. There probably isn't a doctor who hasn't irritated a secretary with an instruction like 'Go back three paragraphs and change *X* to *Z*?' A former supervisor referred to this organising aspect of word processing as 'thought processing'. Some of the techniques we will discuss in this chapter are intended to maximise these organising features.

Recycling, we are told, is good for the biosphere and perhaps also for the infosphere. It's a shame to waste a well-turned phrase and, on many occasions, a little judicious cutting and pasting from existing documents can be quicker than dictating the whole thing afresh.

You may have the best secretary in the world but it won't do you much good if he or she is off sick with winter vomiting virus and the court report is due tomorrow. This would be a very bad time to have to learn the rudiments of word processing!

Finally, if you were lucky enough to qualify for mental health officer status you might soon be in a position to retire and externalise that novel which, we are told, lies within each of us!

Aims and objectives

Modern word processors contain a lot of unused functionality. It is not my intention to try to cover all these capabilities, or even a sizeable proportion of them. Rather, I will discuss a set of under-used features of interest to professional and technical writers. These include styles, outline numbering, tables of contents, outlines, footnotes, templates and collaboration tools.

After reading the chapter I hope that you will be able, for example, to lay out a logical structure for a court report and save it as a template to reuse, or write a scientific paper to match the requirements of a particular journal, or generate an illustrated business plan with feedback and comments from early drafts incorporated into the final version.

Starting standard

I've called this chapter 'Word processing: the next steps' to emphasise that I have aimed it at readers who have mastered the basics of using their computer and are looking to move up to the next step. It is expected that you are able to open and close applications (programs) under your operating system (usually Windows), create and save a word-processed file and do simple editing operations like making words bold, underlining them and so on. If you can't do all these things, it might be sensible to work through the introductory material in Chapter 1.

In this chapter, I mostly use MS Word 97 as an example. This program is several releases behind the latest version of Word but it is still widely used in homes and within the National Health Service. These examples, however, will be equally relevant for those running other versions of MS Word or even other word processors (for example that provided as part of 'OpenOffice', which is freely downloadable from *http://www.openoffice.org*). For those of you following this on Word 2000 (for Windows) or later, however, you may want to disable the 'helpful' adaptive menu feature. Do this by selecting **Tools → Customize → Options**. Untick the **Show Most Recently Used Commands First** box or tick the **Always Show Full Menus** box. Now the menu should stop changing all the time!

If you know that a feature exists and what it might be called, it then becomes a trivial matter to look it up using the help system provided with most programs (from the menu select **Help → Contents** and **Index**) (see Fig. 3.1).

History

Mac Write from Apple is usually credited with being the first WYSIWYG (What You See Is What You Get, pronounced 'wizzywig') word processor and it was introduced to wide acclaim in 1985. Today non-WYSIWYG word

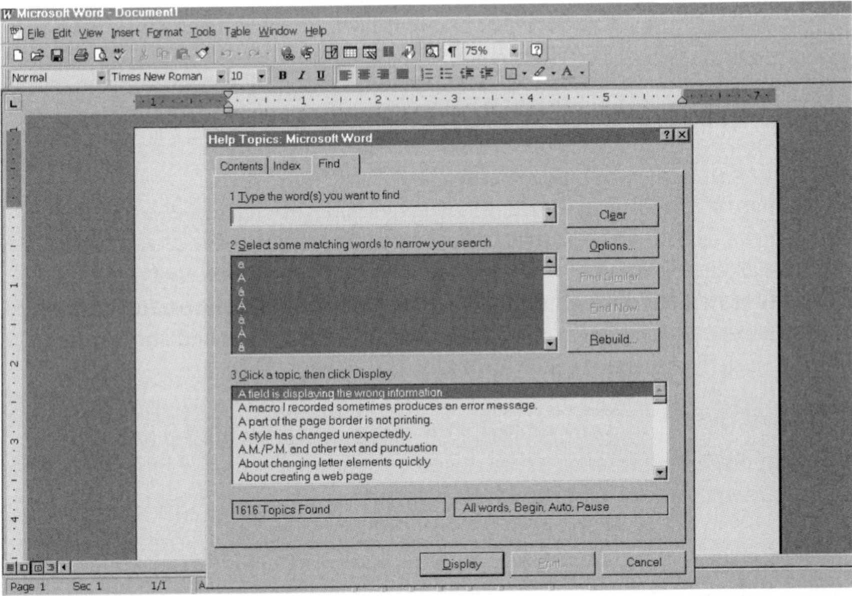

Fig. 3.1 The help system in MS Word.

processors are a rarity and WYSIWYG programs like MS Word are the norm. This may not be an entirely good thing.

WYSIWYG is, at heart, a metaphor: there is an invisible sheet of paper behind the computer screen and the writer is making and erasing marks on this virtual sheet. While superficially attractive, this metaphor seduces the user into wasting time in direct manipulation of the text and can lead him or her to become preoccupied with form over content. Think of how many times you have received a word processed email attachment rich in elaborate fonts and graphics whose content could have been summarised in a few lines of plain text.

A computer is not a typewriter and it can do a lot more than simulate a clattering old Underwood. With a little work, even WYSIWYG programs can be persuaded to take care of many of the low-level formatting tasks, leaving the user free to concentrate on the task of writing itself.

A sense of style

Styles are the basis of many of the automation techniques we discuss below, but they are ignored by a surprising number of computer users. What are paragraph styles? Firstly, what is a paragraph?

On a computer, you make a paragraph by hitting the [RETURN] or [ENTER] key. This terminates the paragraph and starts a new one. Many paragraphs, for example headings, will be only one line long.

Think about the simple editing you've done so far with your word processor, such as choosing different fonts, making text bold or underlined, lining text up in different ways and so on (usually found under the **Format** menu). In addition to this visible formatting, you can specify that the current paragraph is a main heading of your document or a sub-heading or just an ordinary part of the text.

Paragraphs, therefore, have properties, or attributes. A style is just a group of these various properties gathered together and given a name. If you are using MS Word 97, you can see the styles that you've used so far in that document in a box in the top-left corner of the window (Fig. 3.2). To access unused styles, choose the menu item **Format → Style** and in the box titled **List** choose **All Styles** from the drop-down list.

OpenOffice also tries to protect you from too much complexity by only listing the styles you've used so far in a box at the top left of the main window. When starting a new document choose **Format → Stylist** from the menu. In the resulting window (the handy stylist tool) go to the drop-down list at the bottom and choose **All Styles** from the list.

Why use styles?

Not surprisingly, it's a lot quicker to apply a whole group of formatting changes at once via a style rather than piecemeal. More importantly, if you later think all your first-level headings would look better in italicised 12-point Arial rather than 11-point Times New Roman, then you can

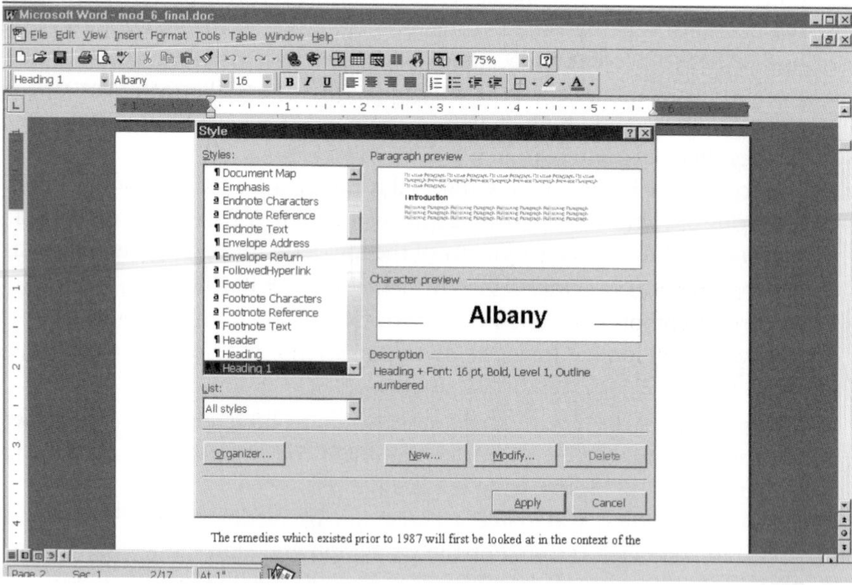

Fig. 3.2 The **Style** dialogue box.

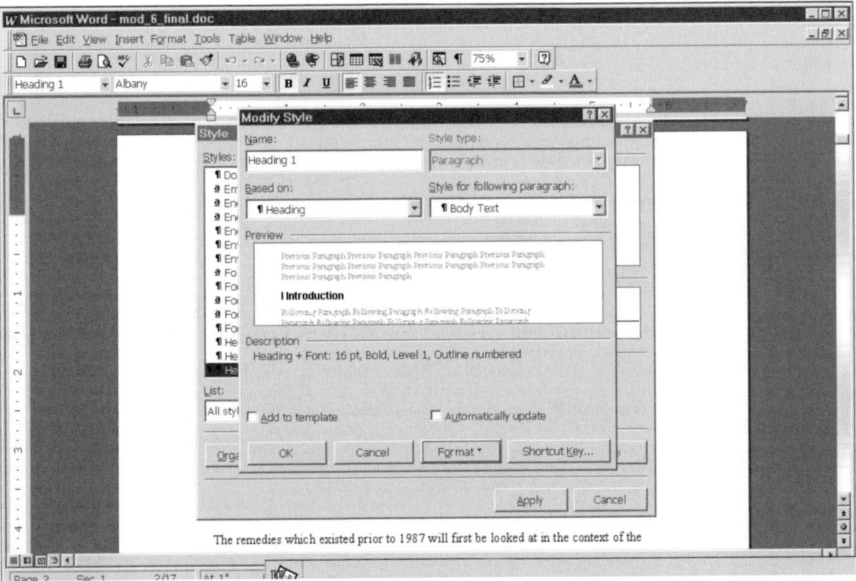

Fig. 3.3 Modifying styles.

simply change the style (see Fig. 3.3) and watch as the computer automatically updates all the parts of the document that used that particular style. Journals differ in their formatting requirements, so careful use of styles means that you can submit a paper to different journals with the minimum of work. In addition to this speed advantage, using styles ensures that all of your headings, titles, ordinary 'body' text and so on look the same throughout your document, giving your work a more professional appearance. Similarly, it looks more professional if all the documents produced by an organisation share a common look and this 'house look' can be enforced by means of styles.

I referred earlier to the use of headings in your document with first-level headings, second-level headings and so on. This is similar to the 'part', 'chapter' and 'section' approach you see in books and reports. Hierarchies get a rather bad press in this postmodern world but for the readers and writers of complex documents they're hard to beat. In the sections that follow, we will look at how this invisible skeleton can be used to automate various tasks, saving you time and effort.

Outline mode

There are those who view the use of outline mode (Fig. 3.4) as being diagnostic of an anankastic personality disorder. I see it as an essential tool for anyone interested in producing complex documents with a rich logical structure, such as court reports or book chapters.

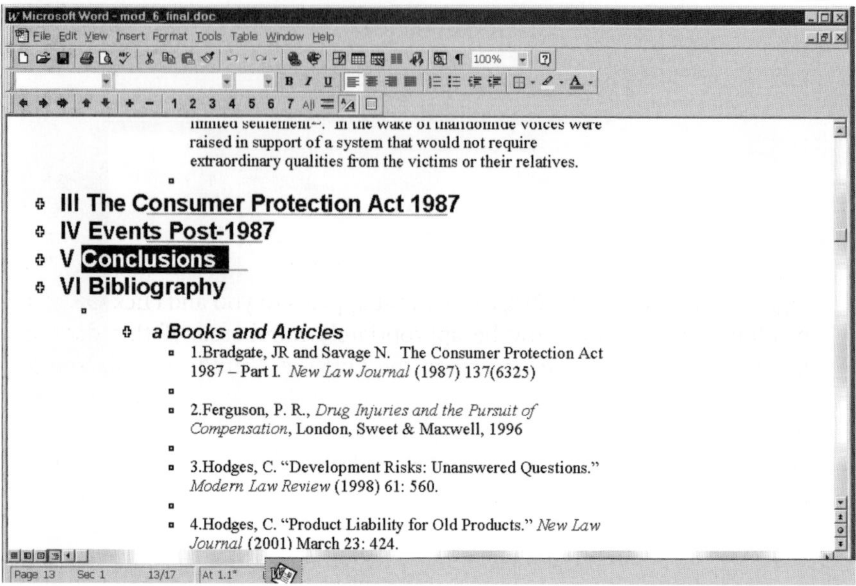

Fig. 3.4 Outline view.

In essence, outline view permits one to see the wood for the trees, selectively to hide the 'ordinary' text of the document so that you can focus on the big picture of headings and sub-headings. Headings can be dragged around to different places or can be 'promoted' or 'demoted', secure in the knowledge that the 'ordinary' text will follow. Note that this will not work if you haven't used styles consistently to begin with.

In MS Word 97 one can access outline mode under the **View** menu. In OpenOffice there is no outline mode as such, although a tool called the navigator fulfils a similar function (**Edit** → **Navigator**).

Outline numbering

While the outline mode may help you as a writer to keep track of your work, the reader will need a similar guide on paper to follow your thinking and, you hope, agree with your conclusions. Therefore, a consistent and logical numbering system is necessary to navigate a printed document of any complexity.

While this could be done manually, you would have to renumber the whole document every time a section was inserted or removed. It is easier to instruct your computer to do this kind of chore. Again, if your computer is to 'know' what number to assign to each section, you will need to have assigned styles to the various parts. If you use the built-in heading styles these should automatically be associated with the appropriate outline level.

Let me give you a word of warning. Outline numbering is notoriously difficult to troubleshoot. I find it much, much easier to set up the numbering *before* writing any text rather than trying to fix it afterwards. Once you have a numbering set-up that works, save it as a template (see below) and reuse it.

First place the cursor in the first top-level heading in the document (e.g. in the heading entitled 'Introduction'). In Word 97, you generate the outline numbers by selecting **Format → Bullets And Numbering**. Click on the **Outline Numbered** tab and various outlining options should appear Fig. 3.5). Select an outlining format that appeals to you and click **OK**. Your heading levels should now be appropriately numbered. If this does not happen you may need to return to the **Outline Numbered** tab, select a format as before but this time click **Customize**. Click on the button marked **More** with two downward pointing arrows to reveal all the options. It may be necessary to link styles manually to outline levels, particularly if you have not used the built-in heading styles. Thus level 1 should link to your top-level heading style ('Heading 1' for example), level 2 to the second-level heading (Heading 2) and so on (Fig. 3.6).

In OpenOffice the process is similar. The relevant functionality is located under **Tools → Outline Numbering**. In the tab that appears you can associate outline number levels with paragraph styles. Start by associating your top-level styles with level 1 in your outline numbering and work downwards through the hierarchy.

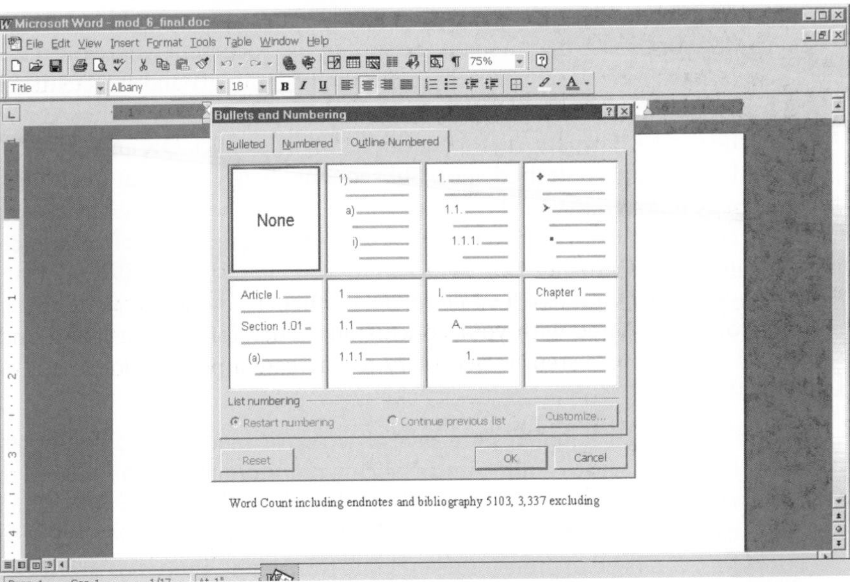

Fig. 3.5 Outline numbering.

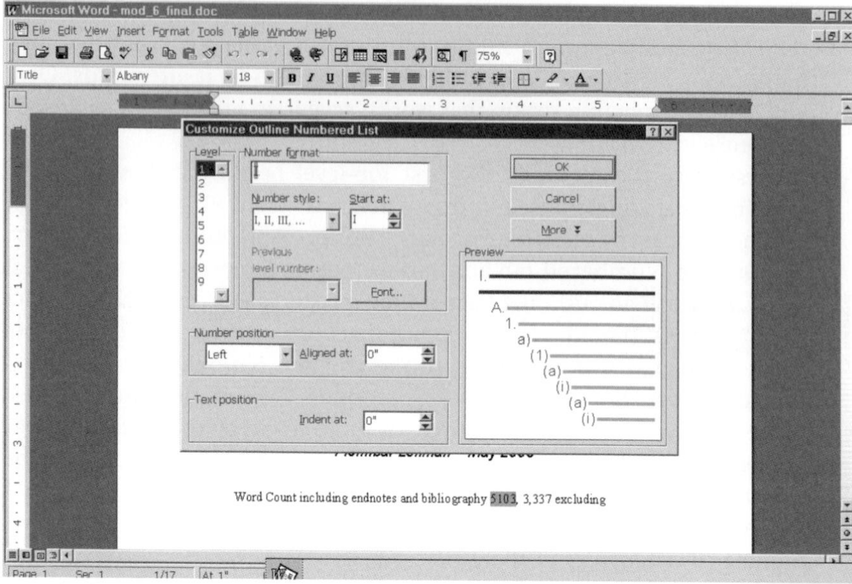

Fig. 3.6 Modifying outline numbering.

Table of contents

A table of contents (TOC) is another navigational tool for your readers. Like outline numbers, this could be done manually but automation yields a more consistent and easily updated result.

In MS Word, place the cursor at the spot in the document where the table of contents is to appear (conventionally the beginning!) and select **Insert → Index and Tables.** Click on the **Table Of Contents** tab and choose one from the various formats on display (Fig. 3.7). Then click **OK** and the TOC should appear at the desired spot. Subsequent changes to your document will not be reflected in your TOC until you click with the right mouse button (right click) anywhere in the TOC. This should bring up a menu from which you can refresh the TOC.

The process is almost identical in OpenOffice.

Templates

In the real world, templates are bits of wood or metal that a craftsman holds back and uses to guide him as he cuts out more bits of the same size and shape. In the more effete world of computing, templates are partial or 'master' documents that are used in a similar way. Just as with real templates, you need to protect the template from being altered so that it can be reused. This could be achieved manually by saving the modified file to a different name but most modern word processors do this automatically.

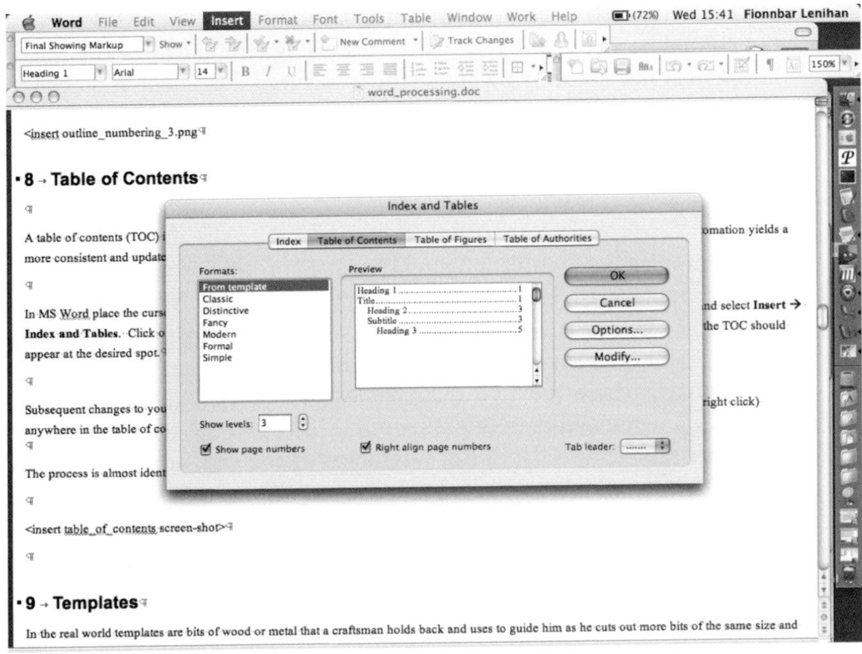

Fig. 3.7 Table of contents.

Templates can contain 'boilerplate' text, formatting, styles, headers, footers and macros (see later). MS Word comes stocked with a wide range of templates that you can see when you choose **New** from the **File** menu. Even a plain blank document is based on a template called *normal.dot*.

Creating your own templates in MS Word is simplicity itself. Just prepare your template as a normal document and when you feel happy with it select **File → Save As**. In the box at the bottom where it says **Save As Type** select **Document Template** from the drop-down list and give your template a meaningful name. Next time you create a new document you will be offered your new template along with the ones MS Word came with.

In OpenOffice you follow a similar procedure to create a template. Make sure to save your template to the *Template* directory under your *OpenOffice.org* directory (on the Windows system I'm using it is *C:\Program Files\OpenOffice.org1.1\user\template*). A wide variety of templates can be freely downloaded from the OpenOffice website.

Recap

In the above sections I have shown you how to provide structure to your documents with styles, how to view and change this structure on screen with outline mode and how to display this structure on paper using outline numbers. In addition to the inherent advantages of a structured document, this approach greatly facilitates the automation of tedious tasks. Finally, I demonstrated how to reuse your hard work using templates.

In the next few sections I will use the structured document as a base to explore other tools that can support you in your writing work.

Referencing

This is a complex field with confusing terms, all of which seem to be based on the names of North American cities (Harvard, Chicago, Vancouver, etc.). James Wooley will be covering the subject of bibliography management in detail in Chapter 8, so we will only touch upon it here.

In summary, there are two main styles of referencing, the Harvard, which uses a name and date (e.g. 'Lenihan, 2003') in the text matched to an alphabetically sorted list of full references at the end, and the numeric Vancouver style, which uses a superscript number corresponding to the number of the full reference listed at the end of a paper or chapter.

For the Harvard style, the use of a package such as Reference Manager, Endnote or Papyrus is recommended. Numeric references have better support in most word processors but the above reference tools still offer significant advantages, such as the ability to download references directly from online databases.

To insert a numeric reference in MS Word (Fig. 3.8) select **Insert → Footnote**. In the box that appears, specify **Endnote** and click **OK**. A

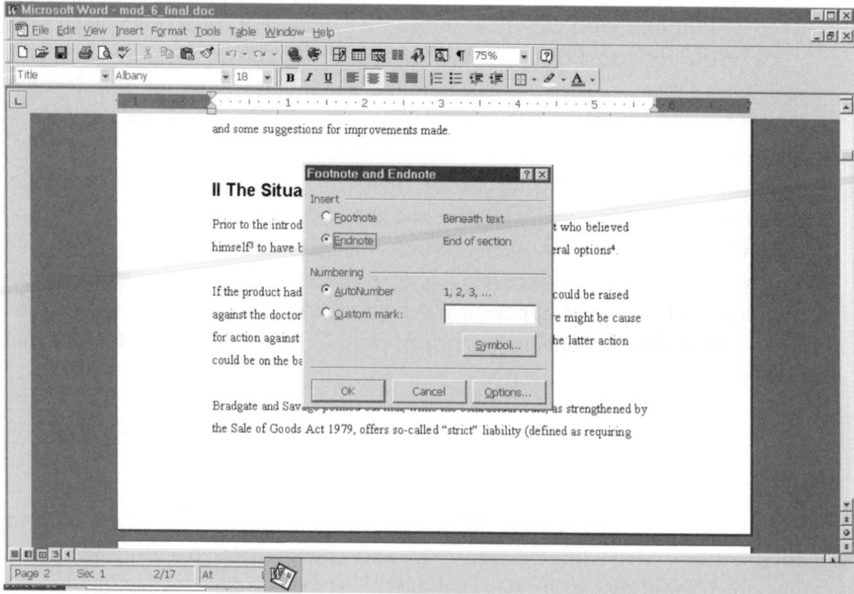

Fig. 3.8 Inserting an endnote.

superscript number will appear at the point where you placed the cursor and you will be taken to a blank line at the end of the document where you can enter the corresponding full reference. OpenOffice works in exactly the same way.

Views

We have tried to convince you of the advantages of moving away from a literal, visual approach to writing towards one based on the logical structure of the document. Nowhere are the advantages of this more evident than in the various 'views' that can be taken of the same document.

We discussed outline mode above. This is perhaps the perspective furthest removed from the printed output. By contrast, print preview is the one that most closely approximates paper. You can access print preview by selecting **File → Print Preview**. In print preview, Word attempts to provide a faithful rendition on-screen of what your printer will produce. The result is a sort of static picture that you cannot modify or edit (though you can print it).

Page layout is selected from the **View** menu and is a sort of print preview in which you can edit the document. Since computer monitors are typically wider than they are long, this wastes space. 'Normal view', in contrast, maximises the amount of editable text on screen but at the expense of looking less like the eventual printed page.

On-line view gives you a so-called 'document map', which is like outline mode on steroids. This too is available from the **View** menu.

Show/hide

If you look along the MS Word toolbar you will come to a button (Fig. 3.9) that looks like some kind of musical notation (usually found to the right). Clicking on this causes little dots to appear between words while the 'musical' symbol marks every new paragraph. You can also access this (on MS Word for Windows) via **Tools → Options → View**.

While initially distracting, the value of marking spaces and paragraphs in this way soon becomes apparent when there are tricky formatting problems that seem to defy rational explanation. OpenOffice has a similar feature that

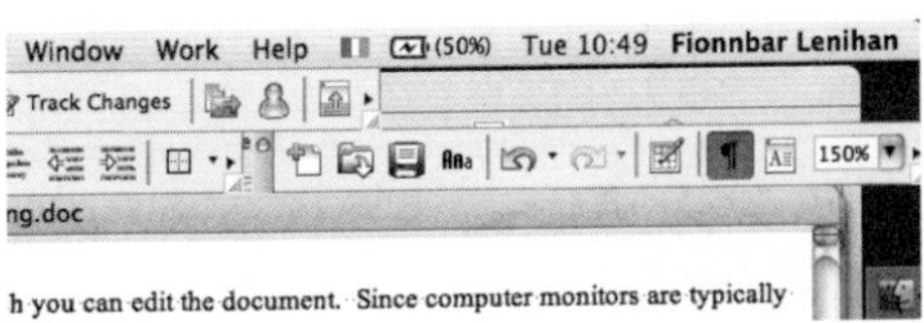

Fig. 3.9 The show/hide button.

is accessed in the same way, while the former market leader WordPerfect went further with its **Reveal Codes** option.

Find/replace

This feature is present in some form in most word processors and text editors. Its sophistication varies between products but the potential of even the simplest version is rarely realised. In most word processors, these functions are found under the **Edit** menu. In MS Word 97, clicking the **More** button at the bottom of the box will bring up advanced features, such as finding formatting or special characters (Fig. 3.10).

One simple trick is to use short abbreviations for words and phrases that are easily misspelled or used inconsistently, perhaps preceded by a character like '|' which one would rarely use. When one has finished writing, a single find and replace changes every occurrence of the abbreviation to the complete (and hopefully correct!) full version.

Find and replace isn't just for regular text: the formatting characters we discussed earlier can be treated in the same way. For example, I often use a three-stage find and replace operation to fix a mangled text file in which every line has been terminated by a single paragraph mark, giving a ragged appearance. 'Real' paragraphs are of course followed by two consecutive paragraph marks. In this case one first needs to protect 'real' paragraphs by replacing them with a little-used character such as a '|'. Now replace all the remaining paragraph marks (which are unwanted) with nothing before

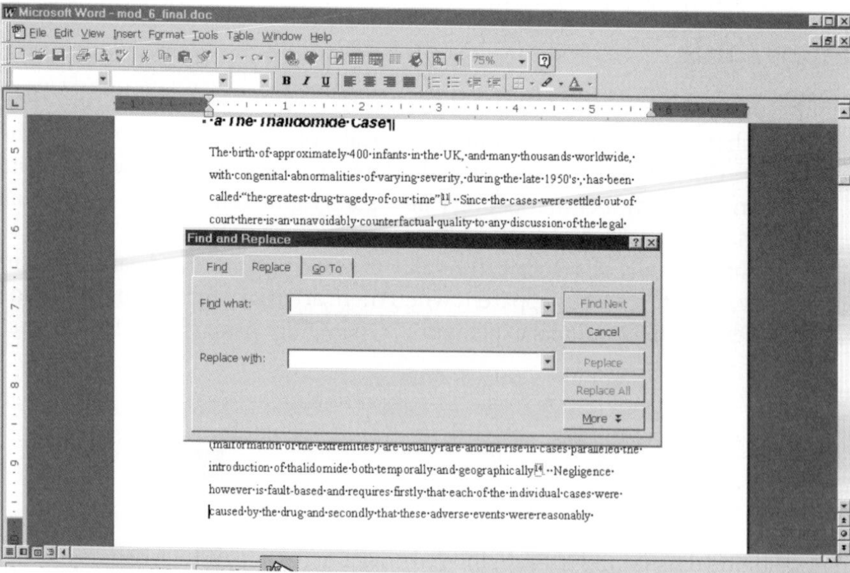

Fig. 3.10 Find and replace.

restoring the 'real' paragraphs by finding every instance of '|' and replacing it with double paragraphs.

For ultimate convenience, this whole sequence could be recorded as a macro and assigned to a keyboard shortcut (see below for macros).

Automation techniques like this can save hours of work, but, of course, the responsibility for the final product remains with the writer, particularly for important documents like court reports.

Headers and footers

Not to be confused with headings, these are pieces of special text which appear at the top (header) or bottom (footer) of every printed page and which can contain constants (text that stays the same) or variables (like page numbers or date of printing).

Even experienced secretaries sometimes use regular text for headers and footers. The problem with this approach is that even minor editing changes can push or pull headers and footers into the middle of the pages, necessitating tedious manual reformatting.

The header/footer feature (Fig. 3.11) lets you create text which, in effect, 'floats' at the top or bottom of each page while the regular text 'flows under it' (this metaphor business is contagious). Normally MS Word and other word processors keep headers and footers invisible during ordinary writing.

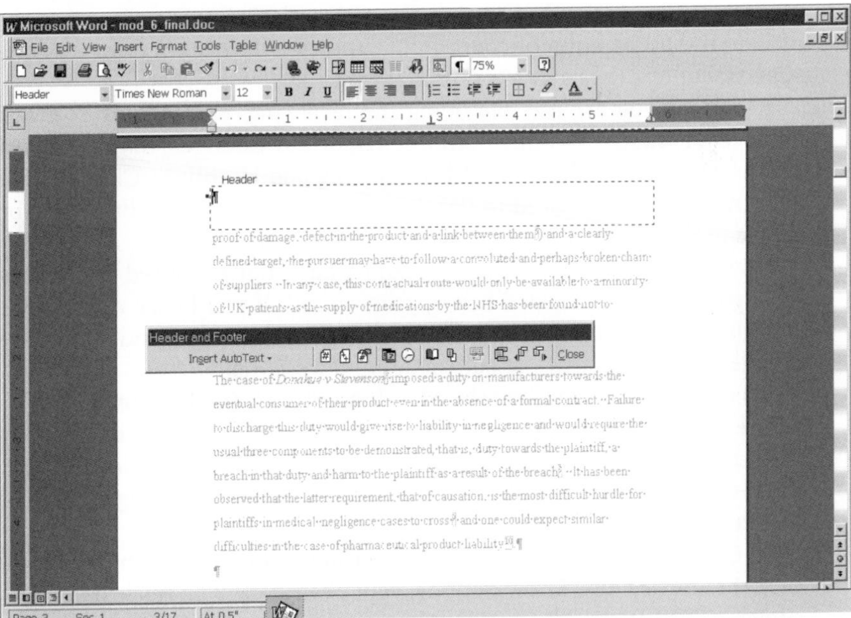

Fig. 3.11 Headers and footers.

Obviously, headers and footers are visible in the printed output and in print preview (though not in page view). They can be edited by selecting **View → Header/Footer**. The constants and variables referred to above can be selected from here. In OpenOffice the corresponding functionality can be accessed by selecting the desired headers directly from the **Insert** menu.

Comments

If you have ever had to edit someone else's work in a non-destructive way (i.e. no red biro) you will have discovered the ever-useful PostIt™ note. This can be replicated *in silico* using MS Word's 'comment' feature. This creates a virtual sticky note which is attached to the document and which travels with it by floppy disk or email. It should not be visible in the final printout unless (for some strange reason) you really want it to be.

This feature can be accessed from the **Insert** menu. The equivalent feature in OpenOffice is called **Note**.

Collaboration

Collaboration, like hierarchy, has a bad name these days. It calls to mind images of shady policemen with moustaches and pillbox hats, bereted resistance fighters and Ingrid Bergman.

More prosaically, it's also the term used to describe features that support multiple authorship and editorship. Examples of this from psychiatry might include the preparation of court and statutory reports by a trainee or the supervision of a thesis by a senior academic.

Assuming you are the one doing the reviewing, go to **Tools → Track Changes**. From the sub-menu, choose **Highlight Changes**. In the box that appears, tick **Track Changes While Editing** and **Highlight Changes On Screen**. You will also need to decide whether you want the changes to be visible in the printed output (I would suggest not).

Now when you delete text it doesn't vanish but has a red line drawn through it. Similarly, added text appears in red. If you hover your mouse over the altered text a pop-up yellow box will give the time and date of the change and the name of the person doing the editing.

When the trainee receives the edited report back (perhaps on disk or by secure internal email), he or she has the option of accepting or rejecting each change individually (by right clicking on the change and selecting from the resulting menu) or globally (by right clicking and selecting **Accept** or **Reject**).

In OpenOffice these tools are located under **Edit → Changes**. If you click the **Record and Show** options, your changes will be tracked in a way similar to MS Word. The recipient goes to the same menu but ticks the **Accept** or **Reject** option.

Graphics and tables

While most journals ask that graphics be submitted as separate files, you may find yourself wanting to embed a picture in a document for an in-house publication such as a report or business plan. To do this, select **Insert → Picture → From File**. Navigate through the file system (see Chapter 1) to the graphic file you want to embed and click **Insert**. There are various kinds of graphic files and should your file be in a format not recognised by your word processor you could easily convert it using tools such as Irfanview (*http://www.irfanview.com*) or the Gimp (*http://www.gimp.org/downloads*).

Clicking once on the newly appeared picture with the left mouse button results in the graphic being selected. It can now be resized and dragged around the page using the mouse.

Continuing with our theme of getting the computer to do all the hard work, if you select **Insert → Caption** (with the picture selected) you will get a chance to attach a label to the new illustration. While this could be done manually, the automatic approach permits you to generate a table of figures in much the same way as the TOC above.

Tables can help clarify (or obscure) a heterogeneous mass of numbers. To create a simple table go **Table → Insert → Table**. **Table → Autoformat** lets you choose an attractive format for the new table.

File formats and exchanging documents

File formats were introduced in Chapter 1. While the MS Word format (denoted by the suffix *.doc*) was given there as a single entity, in reality it has changed over the years to the extent that recent versions of MS Word can have difficulty opening files created by earlier versions. Of course, problems are even more likely in the other direction! The **File → Save As** menu item lets you choose to save a document in the format of an older version of Word or, if you foresee real problems, as a 'rich text format' (*.rtf*) or plain text (*.txt*) file. The latter can be read by almost any word processing program.

File conversions are very likely to disrupt the layout of your document. In some cases, even without file incompatibility, simply moving a file from one computer to another can ruin the appearance of the document, as fonts available on one machine may not match those on another.

For documents that are to be viewed and printed only by the recipient, one interesting option is to convert them to Adobe Acrobat or PDF (Portable Document Format) files. This can be done superbly by the excellent Adobe Acrobat (*http://www.adobe.com*) program or with the free PDF Creator software (*http://sector7g.wurzel6.de/pdfcreator/index_en.htm*). This has the added advantage of eliminating viruses that may be lurking in the Word document (see the section on macros below), reducing the file size and also eliminating hidden information that might be contained in the document.

Macros

Macros are the appropriate place to end our exploration of word processing because a macro is, in essence, a program and with mastery of programming comes the power to add any desired feature. The macro language used in MS Word, Visual Basic for Applications (VBA), is shared across all the MS Office applications and can easily be used to create toolbars and menus just like 'real' parts of MS Office. There are book recommendations at the end of this chapter that should help with getting started in VBA.

Macros can be useful even if you don't aspire to heavy-duty programming. We had the example earlier of a complicated three-step find and replace operation that could easily be automated with a macro. Complex macros require some understanding of programming concepts such as 'loops' and 'variables' but a simple macro can simply be recorded.

While equivalent functionality exists in other programs, MS Word will be used as an example. The macro recorder is accessed using **Tools → Record New Macro** and is represented on-screen by a little box with tape recorder controls (Fig. 3.12). The starting screen gives the option of choosing a combination of keys that can trigger your new creation.

While the recorder is capable of capturing either keyboard or mouse 'events', I have found that using keyboard shortcuts rather than the mouse gives more consistent results. Don't forget to stop the recorder when you have completed the desired actions.

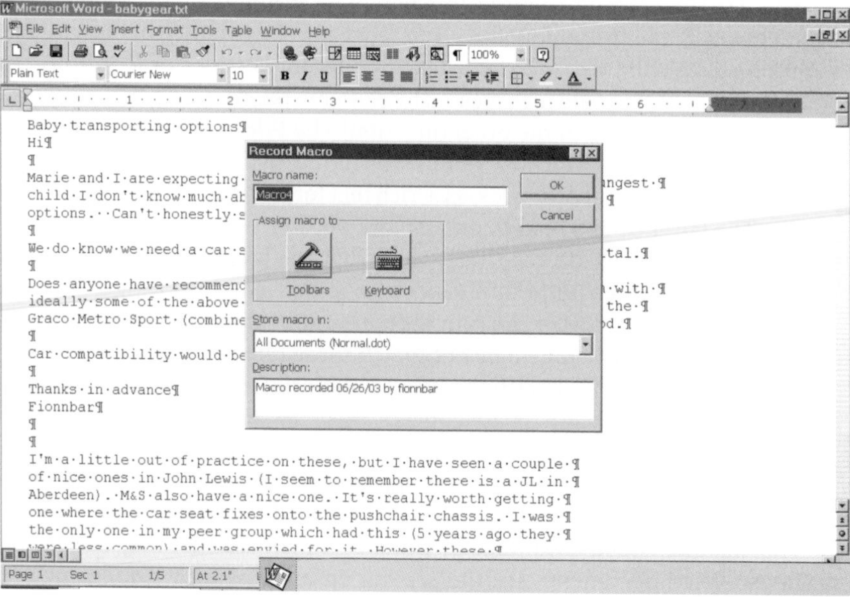

Fig. 3.12 Macros.

Typically, this feature has been abused to create macro viruses. Your copy of Word will warn you if a document contains macros; do not open it if you are not expecting them.

Conclusions

The theme of this book is about taking the next steps with your computer, moving past your initial habits and expectations which, while initially helpful, are now holding you back. In the area of word processing this means seeing past the typewriter metaphor and understanding documents as more than just the printed output. Doing this will free you to produce consistent, highly structured documents rather than amorphous, idiosyncratic blobs of text; it will allow you to automate repetitive tasks and appropriately reuse your own and others' work.

Suggested reading

Hart-Davis, G. (2005) *Word Annoyances: How to Fix the Most Annoying Things About Microsoft Word*. Sebastopol, CA, & Farnham (UK): O'Reilly Media.

Roman, S. (1999) *Writing Word Macros: An Introduction to Programming Word Using VBA* (2nd edn). Sebastopol, CA, & Farnham (UK): O'Reilly Media.

CHAPTER 4

Presentation software

Justine McCulloch

Specialised software has become a necessary part of delivering high-quality presentations. Previous generations of doctors have handed their work over to the medical illustration department to be turned into 35 mm slides or lovingly scripted their own overhead transparencies. No longer. The past decade has seen a seamless, some would argue insidious, transition to the ubiquitous use of presentation software.

Case conferences, journal clubs, undergraduate lectures, postgraduate teaching, induction programmes for senior house officers, in-training assessments, peer group presentations, talks to other professional groups and to patients and carers – the list of occasions where your audience will expect you to use presentation software is ever growing. Whether you choose to fulfil such expectations is a cost–benefit analysis only you can make for yourself. However, compliance does reap certain rewards: your audience is not unsettled by your non-conformity at the outset; you will increase your chances of looking professional; you have a concrete structure to use as the basis of your presentation; at least some members of your audience will concentrate on your presentation software rather than staring unnervingly at you for the duration of your talk; some information is far easier to impart in the visual than in the auditory modality; if you lose your train of thought a seamless recovery is much more likely; and you will easily be able to generate a handout to give your audience, which removes their need for note-taking and therefore wins approval before you have uttered your first word.

A few words of caution

However, the product remains only as good as the craftsman and when it comes to the quality of the presentations we create, the difference between a good presentation and a great one seldom comes down to software.

It is worth bearing in mind that presentation software was designed for business use and it generally fits imperfectly into the field of medicine. Detractors, such as Susan Dunn of Frugalmarketing.com, would argue that presentation software is often over-used, can be confusing or a crutch for the presenter's insecurity, and often masks poor content. She goes on to point out that a poorly designed presentation can overload the audience or, worse, lull them to sleep.

Edward Tuft, author of several books on the visual display of information, is another such detractor. He is a particularly vigorous critic of PowerPoint (PP):

'As consumers of presentations … you should not trust speakers who rely on the PP cognitive style. It is likely that these speakers are simply serving up PowerPointPhluff to mask their lousy content.'

He bemoans the fact that such presentations do not use grammatical English, that the information on each slide is so sparse that excessive numbers of slides are needed; a 'relentless sequentiality' results and understanding context and evaluating relationships are thereby made more difficult. He also makes the point that the medium is not appropriate for certain types of information:

'Consider … a table of survival rates for those with cancer relative to those without cancer for the same time period. Some 196 numbers and 57 words describe survival rates and their standard errors for 24 cancers.'

He calculates that applying the PowerPoint templates to this information would explode it into six separate 'chaotic' slides, consuming 2.9 times the area of the table.

For a more light-hearted view on the limitations of PowerPoint see Peter Norvig's website (*http://www.norvig.com/Gettysburg/*), which recasts Abraham Lincoln's famous speech as a PowerPoint presentation.

However, the eclectic and discerning medic can use PowerPoint as a tool to create visually attractive slides that form the underpinning of a presentation. The challenge of keeping your audience awake over the whirr of the machine and the progression of the slides may remain, but there is no reason to serenade them to sleep with the hum of your voice reading slide after slide. Successful presentations use presentation software as a tool, not a crutch.

Perhaps George Mallory's aphorism forms a salutary warning: using a feature 'because it's there' may find you lost on a metaphorical Everest in the middle of your presentation. Not all information is easily conveyed in bullet points, which are intended to persuade, not necessarily to convey the truth. Your audience may look for the hidden message even when there isn't one. You may also find presenting the information you need frustrating given the limitations of the format, particularly where the devil really is in the detail. The tenet of 'because it's there' is also best avoided when considering galleries of clip art, transition effects, chart types and the shapes used for bullet points. For most medical presentations such effects should be used sparingly (if at all): it's time consuming to use them, and they will distract some of your audience, irritate others and detract from the overall message.

Aims and objectives of the chapter

Presentation software and computerised presentations are often referred to generically as 'PowerPoints' but in fact the PowerPoint package is only one, albeit very popular, option. We will briefly discuss these alternatives before walking you through the creation of a simple presentation in PowerPoint. There then follow 'window dressing' tips and presention pointers, other tools, some presentation tips and further resources.

Presentation software

There are many presentation graphic programmes to choose from: PowerPoint, Freelance, Corel Presentations, Keynote (for Mac) and most importantly OpenOffice for Windows, Mac and Linux.

We also cover OpenOffice in the word processing and spreadsheet chapters (3 and 5, respectively). This is a completely (and legally) free program which can be downloaded from *http://www.openoffice.org* or ordered on CD by clicking the link at *http://distribution.openoffice.org/cdrom/*. OpenOffice has most of the commonly used features of PowerPoint and can read and write PowerPoint files as well as its own data format.

Creating your first presentation

PowerPoint has a particularly detailed 'wizard' (or automated helper) which handles the basics of creating a presentation. The autocontent wizard (Fig. 4.1) walks you through the type of presentation you want to give; options include 'generic', 'brainstorming', 'communicating bad news' (this approach is best avoided in the clinical setting!) and so on. You then decide what format you want your presentation to be in (i.e. on-screen presentation, web presentation, black-and-white overheads, coloured overheards or 35 mm slides). The third step is to fill in your title and on completion the software produces a list of slides and tells you what areas to cover on each.

Alternatively, if you know what you want to say and want some freedom of expression to do so, clicking on **Blank Presentation** or **From Design Template** will give you this. With the former you even get to design your own slides for that added touch of individuality.

Once you have created your presentation file the first slide automatically comes up as the title slide on which to introduce yourself and your topic. Further slides, added using the menu item **Insert → New Slide**, tend to appear as a small header box and a larger lower text box (Fig. 4.2). You can change this and use different text and content layouts by selecting the menu item **Format → Slide Layout** (Fig. 4.3). You can also change the size of the boxes by clicking and dragging them to the size of your choice. For

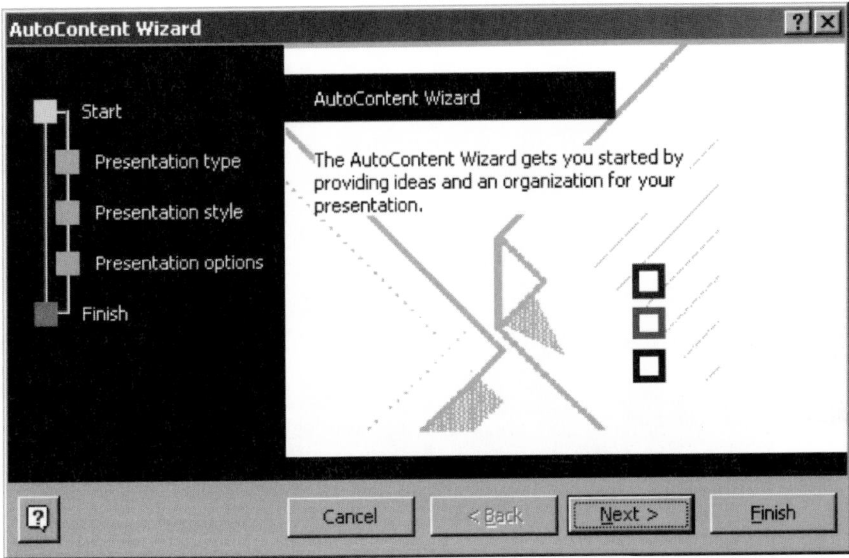

Fig. 4.1 PowerPoint autocontent wizard.

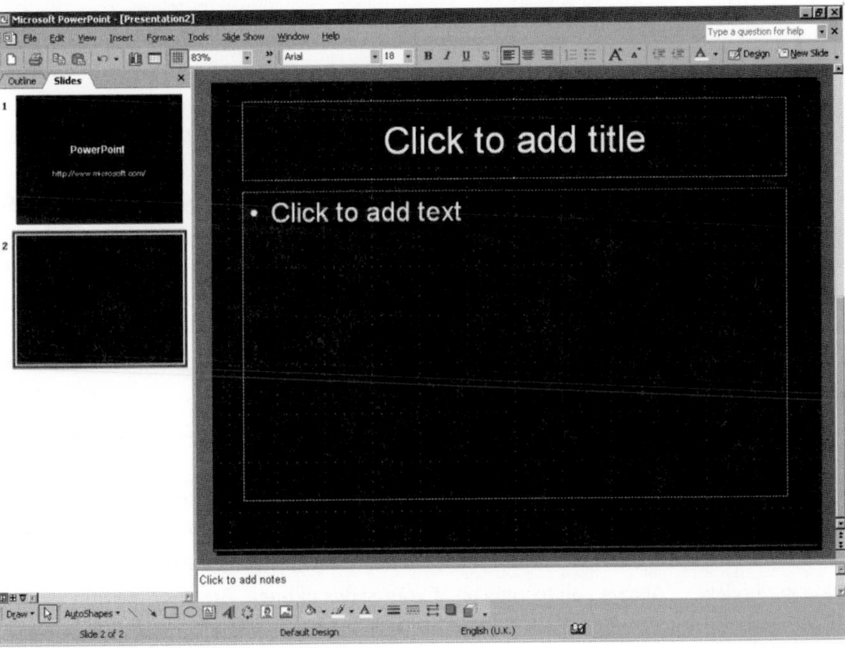

Fig. 4.2 Inserting additional slides in PowerPoint.

anyone prone to this, the grid (**View → Grids And Guides**) makes a handy tool for alignment. This is only available within 'normal' or 'notes' page views. There are six different views found in PowerPoint (see Table 4.1);

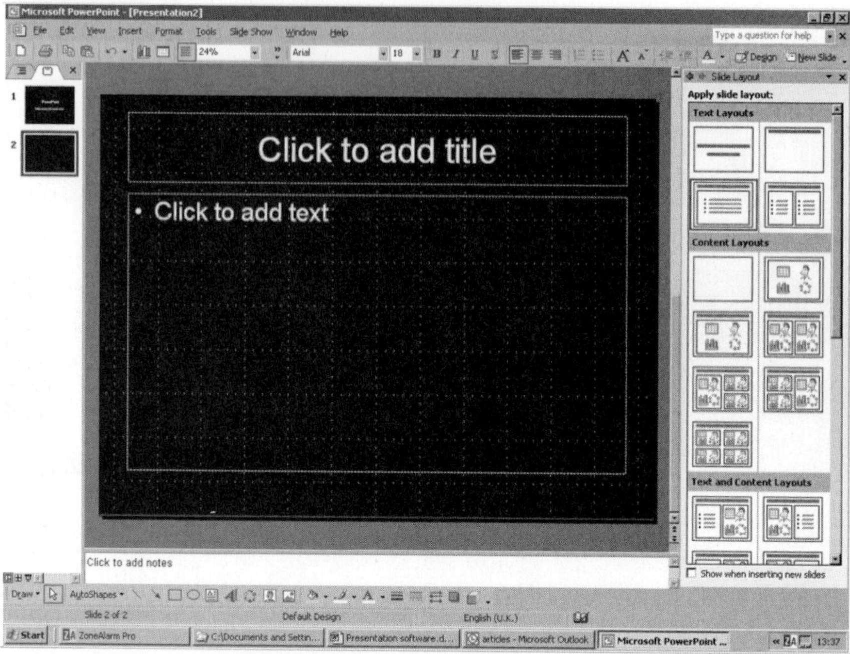

Fig. 4.3 Slide layout.

the default is the 'normal' view. The six views and what they are best used for are shown below. These are accessed from the menu item **View**.

To start writting your presentation, simply follow the on-screen instructions and **Click to add text**. PowerPoint offers a range of fonts, and text can be bold, underlined or italicised (Fig. 4.4); there are also different alignments, and bulleting and numbers can be changed to the format you prefer. However, this can prove time wasting and it is invariably preferable

Table 4.1 PowerPoint view

View name	Note
Normal view	Triple-pane view. You can view the notes, outline and slide all at once
Slide view	Best used when working on your slides individually. The majority of the screen space is for your slide, which allows easier viewing
Slide sorterview	Allows you to view all of your slides at once. Great for moving slides around and deleting or just looking at the flow of your show
Outline view	Best for working on adding your text for the show. Work in an outline format
Notes page view	View a small image of the slide along with space to write your speaker notes
Slide show	This is for previewing and actually running the show. The slides will be full screen

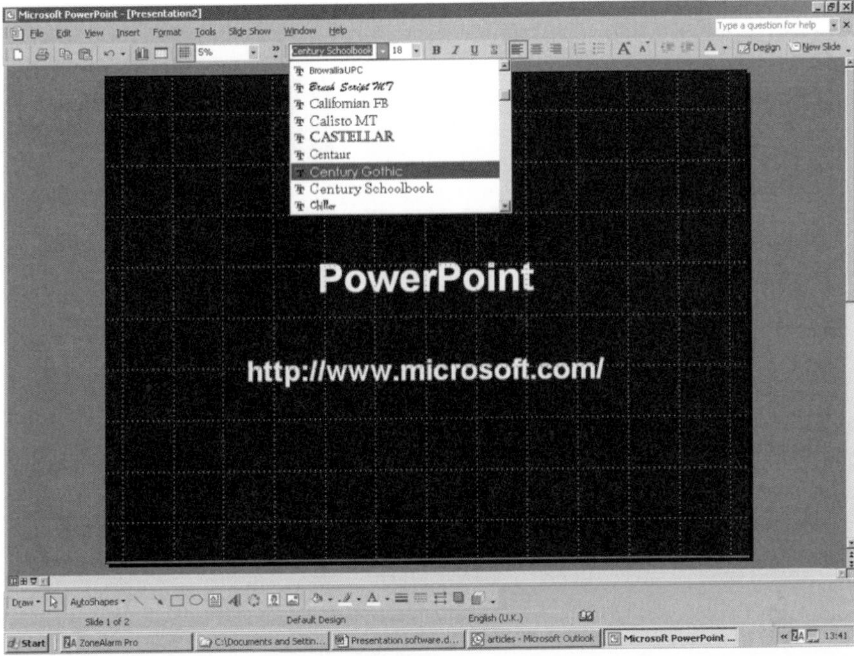

Fig. 4.4 'Word processing' – formatting text in PowerPoint.

to address the content of the presentation and then attend to the aesthetics later, as we will do here.

Unless you are phenomenally well organised, at some point you will probably decide that the content would be clearer or the presentation flow better if you delivered your slides in a different order. This can be done by clicking and dragging from the normal view; however, it is easier to do in the slide sorter view (Fig. 4.5). This also allows you to take an overview of the presentation and check the clarity of your argument.

Another handy tool is the **Hide Slide** command (Fig. 4.6), especially if you decide to 'tweak' the talk at the last minute but don't want to delete slides or start to transfer them to another file.

Aesthetics

'Clothes make the man. Naked people have little or no influence on society.' (Mark Twain)

The same is true of PowerPoint presentations.

'Fashions fade; style is eternal.' (Yves Saint Laurent)

Also true of PowerPoint presentations.

'Fashion is a form of ugliness so intolerable that we have to alter it every six months.' (Oscar Wilde)

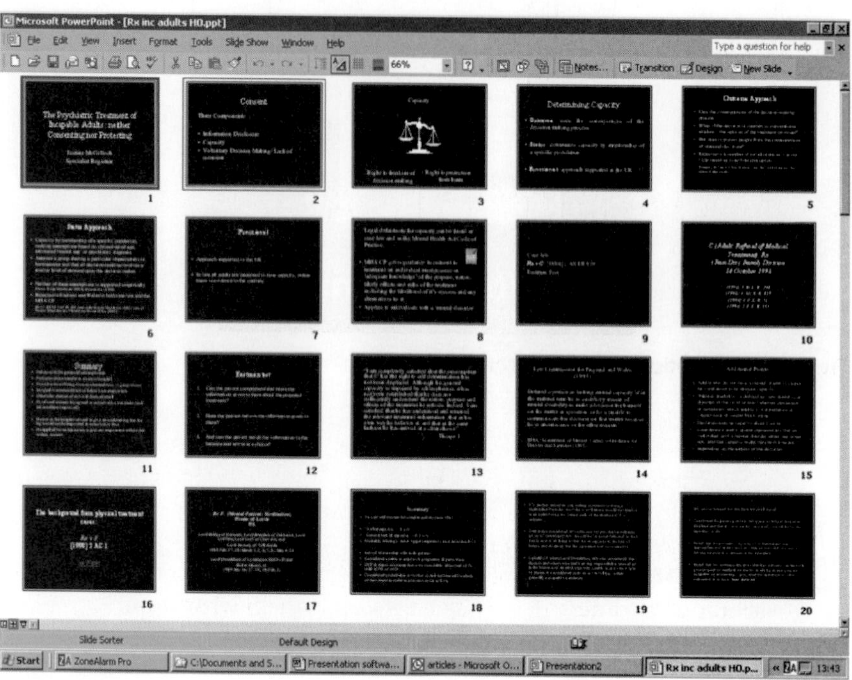

Fig. 4.5 Slide sorter view.

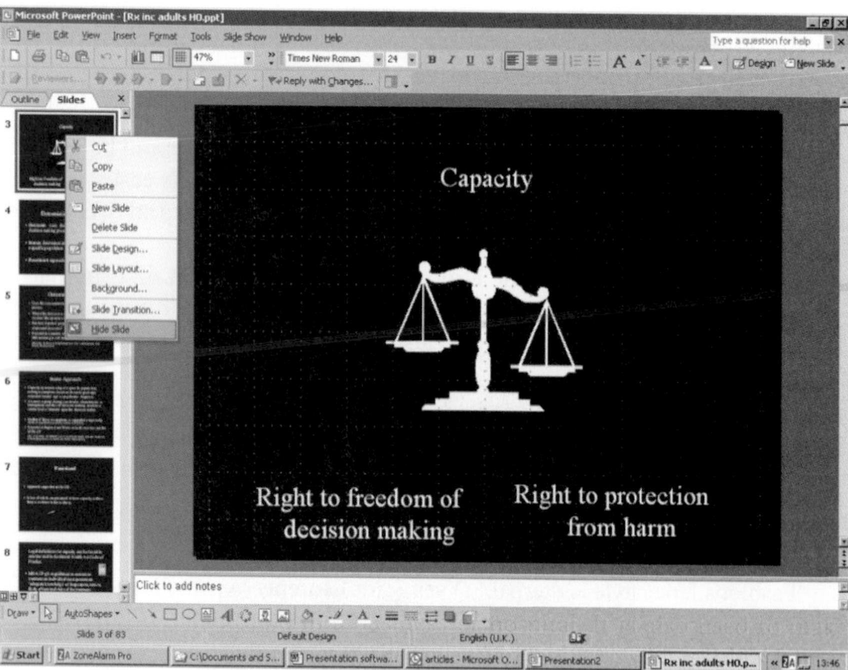

Fig. 4.6 Hide slide.

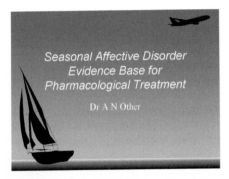

Fig. 4.7 Presentation detracting from content.

Unfortunately, there is no definitive guide to style versus fashion in PowerPoint. You will have to judge for yourself. However, the following might be useful to bear in mind.

First, does the appearance detract from the message (Fig. 4.7)? Show the presentation to different people and then ask them what the most striking thing was and what they thought the take-home message was. If you don't like the answers, change the presentation.

Second, there are some things other people find irritating: the author's personal pet hate is anything that takes longer to materialise on the screen than the time needed to blink. The animation schemes under the 'exciting' heading are a particular source of angst.

Third, a key consideration is whether the text can be easily read (Fig. 4.8). Is the colour scheme such that the text stands out? Is the font big enough to read but not so big that the slide looks as though it belongs in a book for young readers?

Fourth, is there a manageable amount of information on the slide? If it is too busy the audience won't bother to read it.

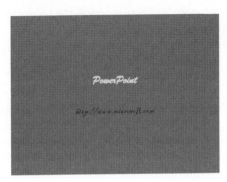

Fig. 4.8 Example of a slide on which font, text size and colours reduce readability.

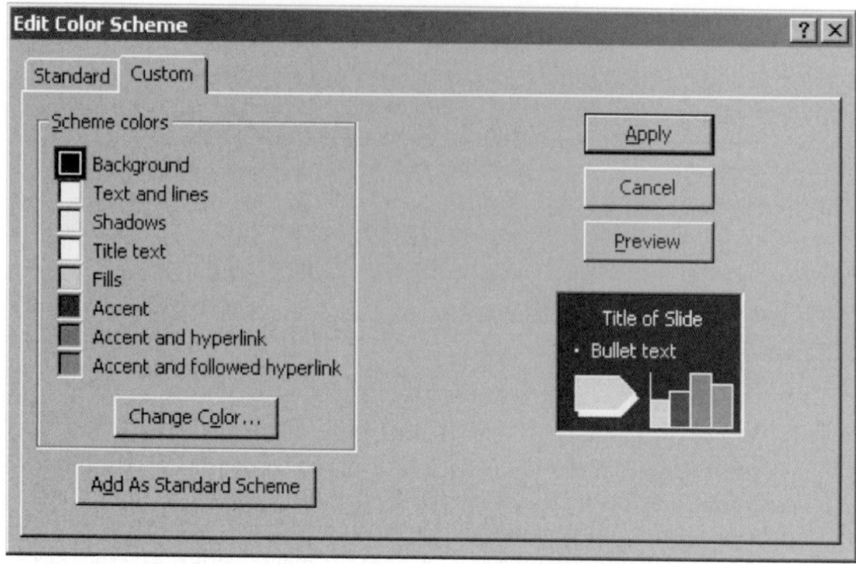

Fig. 4.9 Design your own slides.

Fifth, you should aim for around one slide for every minute of your presentation.

Finally, make sure you have spell-checked your presentation; also make sure the spell-checker has not auto-corrected some professional jargon, turning the sentence into gibberish.

If you choose not to use a design template, then you will need to decide on a background (Fig. 4.9). This is done by accessing the menu item **Format → Slide Design → Colour Schemes → Edit Colour Schemes → Apply.** Probably the best thing to do is to play around with the different effects and see what suits your taste. This is also the time to change fonts and fine-tune the presentation.

The author makes no apology for her views on animation effects; however, if you must go down this route, the relevant options are found under **Slide Show** on the menu.

Other tools

Images and multimedia clips, on the other hand, can work extremely well. You can import pictures, sound (e.g. CD tracks) and movie clips by accessing the **Insert** command and then the appropriate action (Fig. 4.10).

Pictures from other sources can be reformatted to the appropriate size by clicking on the imported picture and then selecting the **Format Picture** option (Fig. 4.11), which allows the size, position, colour and so on to be

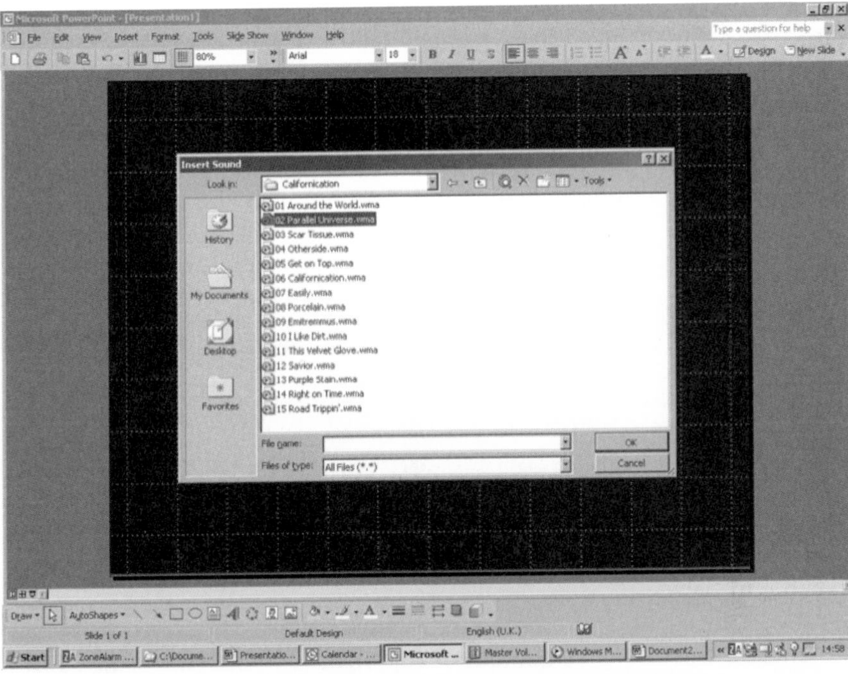

Fig. 4.10 Inserting a sound file into a presentation slide.

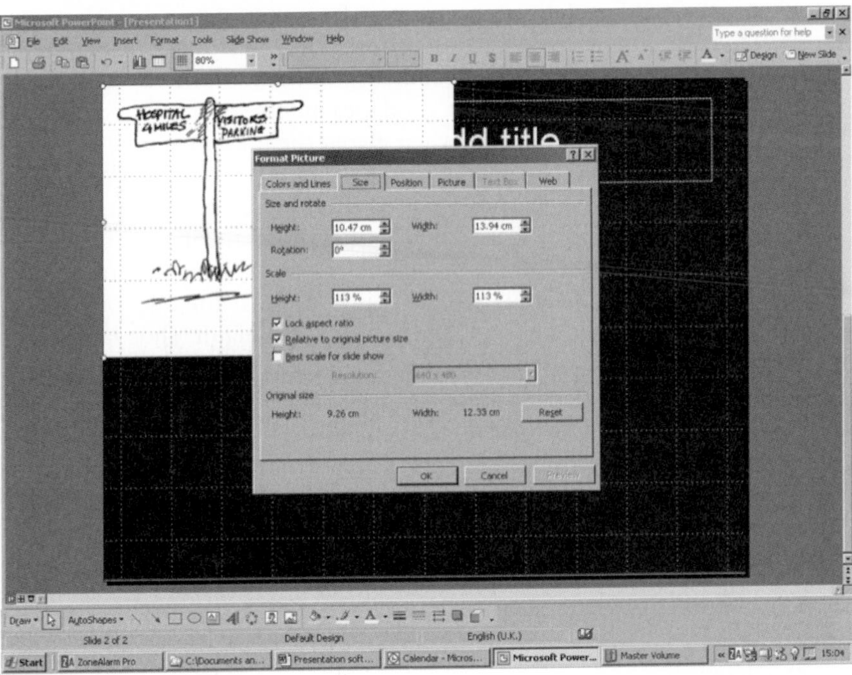

Fig. 4.11 Format pictures.

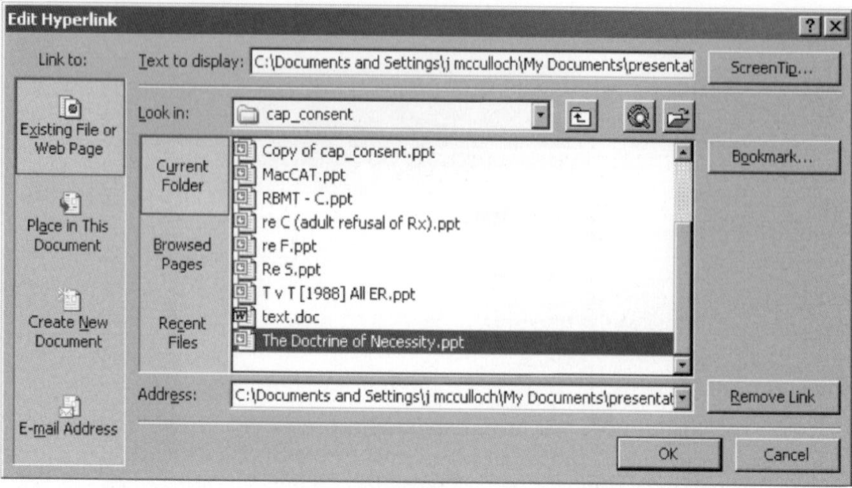

Fig. 4.12 Hyperlinks.

altered. Obviously, be mindful of copyright law when importing. David Harris discusses copyright and other legal matters in Chapter 12.

Another useful tool is the hyperlink, which allows greater flexibility when presenting and gives the option of expanding on particular areas or not, as the audience dictates. This too is accessed under **Insert** on the menu and you can link to any document you wish (Fig. 4.12). Obviously, hyperlinking to a website is not a good idea unless you are confident there will be the facility to be online when giving the presentation.

It is also possible to convert MS Word documents into PowerPoint presentations and visa versa, using the **File** → **Send To** menu item in both programs. You will likely have to do some manual tidying afterwards.

In addition, PowerPoint is a flexible medium in which to prepare poster presentations (Fig. 4.13). This involves just the one, or possibly two, slide(s) which you format as you wish. By default, slide layouts are set up for landscape orientation. However, most posters are prepared in portrait. To change the slide orientation access the **File** menu, **Page Setup** → **Orientation for Slides** → **Portrait.**

Audience notes and handouts are easily prepared by changing the **View** → **Slide Sorter** and then accessing **File** → **Print Preview** → **Slides** → **Handouts** (*x* slides per page) (Fig. 4.14). How the different handouts will look can be previewed via **View** → **Master** → **Handout Master.**

All that remains is to save and close your newly created presentation. PowerPoint can also be saved in HTML format (Chapter 10) or as a self-contained executable file for computers that do not have the programme installed.

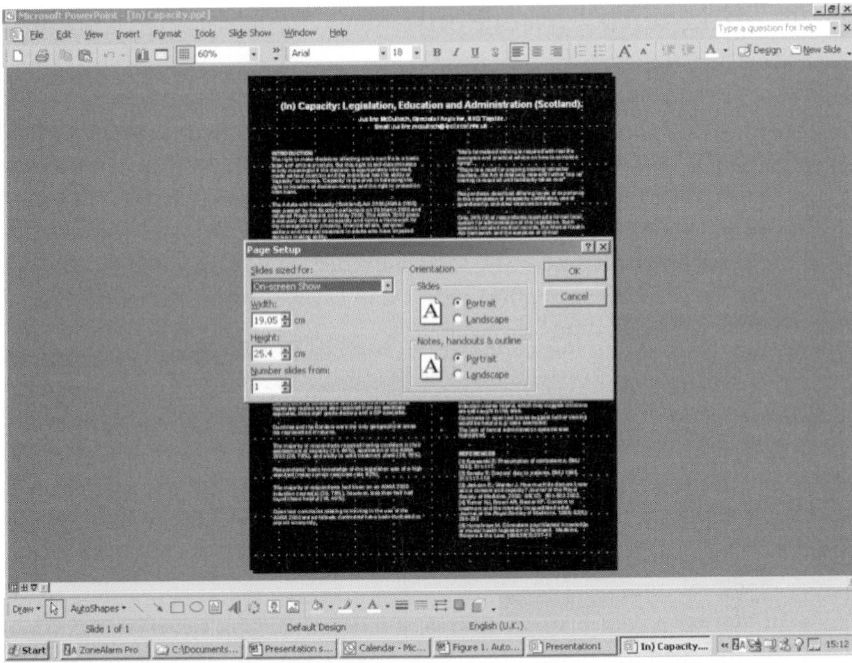

Fig. 4.13 Poster presentations.

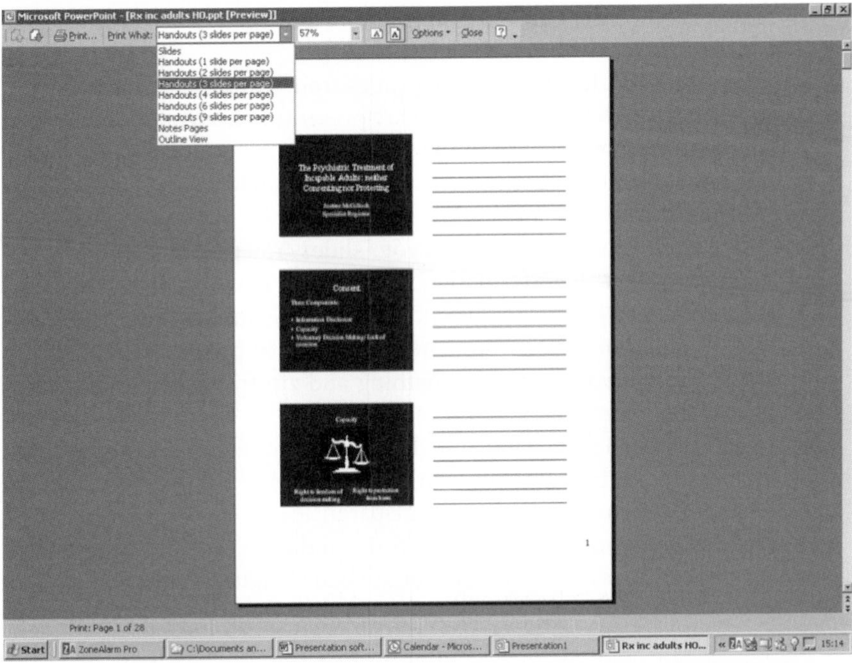

Fig. 4.14 Handouts.

Presenting with PowerPoint

The golden rules of presenting do not change just because you have used presentation software. These are:

- appear practised and at ease
- don't read your talk
- speak at a reasonable rate – not too fast or slow
- speak clearly and audibly – don't mumble
- use the time allotted effectively – don't run short or over the allotted time, and leave time for discussion.

In addition the following may be helpful:

- Check your presentation is working before you stand in front of your audience.
- If you have sent it to someone else and it is on an unfamiliar machine make certain you can navigate your way around.
- If you have brought your own laptop make sure it is connected up in plenty of time.
- If you have your presentation on a USB stick, check everything works on the alien machine.
- A trial run at any 'foreign' venue is invaluable.
- If your physiological tremor tends to become pathological when in front of an audience, rest on something and steady your hand if you need to use the cursor.
- If you have a gadget for changing slides from a distance, make sure it is compatible with the machine you are presenting from and that it hasn't suddenly died on the way to the presentation.
- If you do use such a gadget for changing slides, beware the physiological tremor if clicking on a hyperlink, for example.
- Give people enough time to read your slides. You prepared them, so you must think that the information they contain is worth knowing.
- Be prepared to go backwards and forwards if your audience needs you to (this shouldn't generally be necessary but be prepared to do so).
- Don't panic if you lean on something and zip through five slides in a nanosecond; just smile -and reverse back.
- In addition, rehearse what you are going to do if your equipment fails. Be prepared to talk without your presentation or bring a backup in the form of handouts or overhead transparencies.
- Last but most important, speak to the audience, not the computer or the projection screen. Use appropriate body language. Try to gauge how your audience is responding and fine-tune your presentation to their needs.

Conclusion

Remember, presentation software is there to help you appear slick and knowledgeable. You control it; neither Microsoft nor any other provider controls you! And there is nothing to be frightened of – other than your audience, of course!

Further resources

http://www.med.fsu.edu/informatics
http://www.evsc.k12.in.us/icats/present/classroom.htm
http://office.microsoft.com/en-us/FX010857971033.aspx
http://www.bitbetter.com/powerlinks.htm
http://www.frugalmarketing.com/dtb/powerpoint-kill.shtml
http://exwww.wired.com/wired/archive/11.09/ppt2.html
http://www.inc.com/magazine/20030801/ahanft.html

CHAPTER 5

Spreadsheets

Karen Tingay

The aim in this chapter is to give a brief overview of the use of a spreadsheet package, using as examples both Microsoft Excel and Calc, the free spreadsheet program included in OpenOffice. We will take the reader through the basics of spreadsheets, then move on to look at how this type of program can be used in routine clinical practice. The former section is aimed at people who have never used a spreadsheet package before. Readers familiar with programmes like Excel or Calc may wish to skip that section and go straight to the example. You can follow the examples using Excel, which is part of Microsoft Office (see *http://www.informatics.nhs.uk/cgi-bin/item.cgi?id=703* for a cheap deal on this software for National Health Service employees; alternatively you can download the free OpenOffice software from *http://www.openoffice.org*).

For those of you following this on Excel 2000 (for Windows) or later, you may want to disable the 'helpful' adaptive menu feature. This can be done by selecting **Tools** → **Customize** → **Options**. Untick the **Show Most Recently Used Commands First** box.

What is a spreadsheet?

A spreadsheet is a table in which you can enter data that you wish to analyse. Data are organised in rows and columns with headings to help you make sense of it all. You can manipulate the data to answer whatever questions you may have, for example by sorting fields from highest to lowest, calculating averages and other mathematical functions, or filtering your spreadsheet to show only particular values. You can also create a wide variety of graphs.

Macros can also be used to automate repetitive work. Detailed instruction in writing macros is beyond the scope of this chapter but the 'help' facility of your spreadsheet program will get you started.

What can I do with a spreadsheet?

Spreadsheets are usually associated with high-powered financial types and it is true that the first ones were developed for this sector. However, any information that has a list, or table-like, quality is amenable to a spreadsheet approach. Some examples are given below.

In your personal life, a spreadsheet can keep a running total of your exercise regimen, weight lost and calories expended, with pretty graphs showing (you hope) progress towards your goals. Such a system would also have interesting clinical applications, given recent interest in medication-induced weight gain and metabolic side-effects.

In teaching, spreadsheets are often used to maintain attendance lists, examination results, grades, lesson plans and timetables.

In administration, spreadsheets are a life-saver for those unfortunates who have the task of developing on-call and shift rotas, since running totals of various types can easily be generated and compliance checked more easily.

A spreadsheet is no substitute for a proper database (see Chapter 6) but it can be enough for simple data collection and analysis. It can be particularly useful for 'cleaning up' data exported from another program, for example preparing an address list to use in a mail merge or mass mailing. Spreadsheets typically have better charting abilities than databases, which is why many database users export their data into a spreadsheet for this purpose.

Similarly, while spreadsheets are no substitute for dedicated statistical data analysis programs like SPSS or R (see Chapter 7), they are probably easier to use for simple descriptive statistics.

You may not be a high-powered financial type but you will probably have to deal with budgets or business plans at some point and the ability to work a spreadsheet will probably then be essential.

We hope the above examples have convinced you that the spreadsheet should find a place in your armamentarium, whether you are a teacher, manager, researcher or 'just' a clinician. For the rest of this chapter we will work through one possibility, that of a clinician who wishes to evaluate or audit her own work.

The basics

Some terms

If you have never used a spreadsheet before, there are a few terms you may not have come across. You may find it useful to have a blank Calc or Excel spreadsheet open during this section.

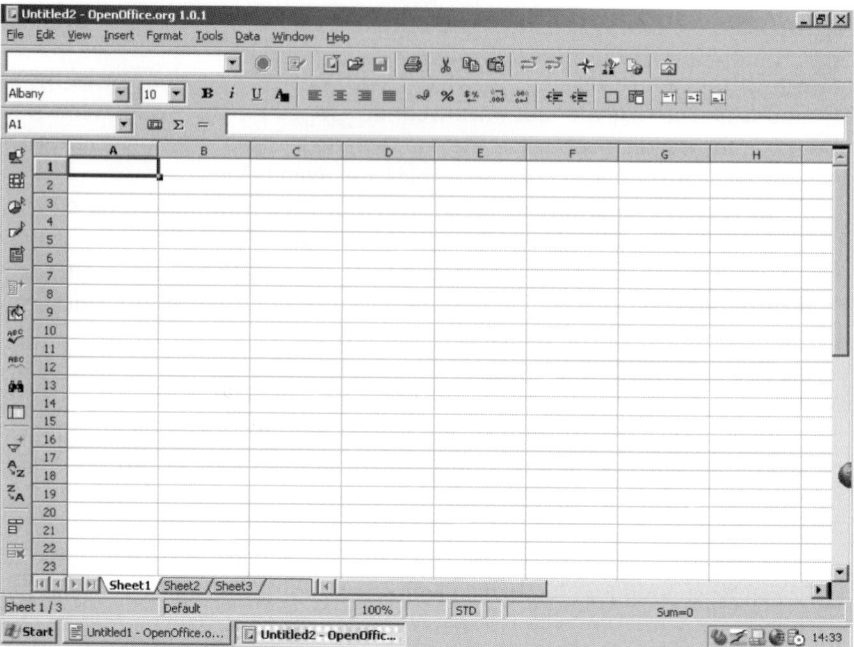

Fig. 5.1 An empty OpenOffice Calc screen.

- A *sheet* is the spreadsheet you happen to be working on at that particular time. By default, at the bottom of the screen are three tabs, labelled sheets 1–3 (Fig. 5.1). These can be useful if you want to include similar but separate data in the same file. For example, a clinician may wish to audit her work in 6-monthly increments and may choose to separate the information by using different sheets. Alternatively, the clinician could use these other sheets to store graphs that might otherwise clutter up the original sheet. We recently used different sheets when describing different aspects of a data-set to make it easier for those commenting on the work to make sense of it. In this instance, the sheets were named according to the data fields being represented, such as 'Demographic data', 'Referral data', 'Clinical data', and so on.
- A *workbook* is the spreadsheet document consisting of all your sheets, graphs, macros and formulae.
- A *cell* is one of the individual elements making up the spreadsheet. Cells typically hold data or formulae but can also be used for just labelling columns, for example.

Opening Calc

On opening OpenOffice Calc, you see the screen shown in Fig. 5.1. At the very top of the screen you can see the menu bar; directly under that is the

Table 5.1 Keys used to navigate around spreadsheets

Key(s)	Movement of cursor
Tab	Next cell to the right
Shift + tab	Back one cell
←	Back one cell
↑	Up one cell
→	Next cell to the right
↓	Down one cell

function bar, with commands like **Open**, **Save**, **Copy** and **Paste**. Below that is the object bar, which, by default, contains formatting options. To the side is the main tool bar, which contains commands for inserting files, finding particular entries, filtering and sorting, and so on. Holding the mouse pointer over any of the command buttons displays their title.

Moving around the sheet

You can move from cell to cell using the mouse or keyboard. Clicking from cell to cell using your mouse is time consuming and can be problematic if your cells are small. Much easier, then, to use the tab or arrow keys on the keyboard. Table 5.1 shows the different key combinations you can use to navigate your way around.

Moving between sheets in a workbook

You may have related data that cannot be included with the rest of the information. The clinician in our example might want to separate out-patients from different groups or records. As long as the data in each different group is not intended to be merged it works well to use different sheets.

Types of data

Spreadsheets allow for different types of data to be entered – for example, Number, Percent, Currency, Date, Time, Fraction, Scientific, Boolean, Text, or User-Defined. Each allows different formats to be applied so that the data displayed and used will be of the most value to the user. These data types will be explained in more detail in Chapter 6, on databases.

Formatting cells

Cells can be formatted in exactly the same ways as text documents. You can change the font, font size, style, colour, background colour, lines, and so on. It is worth experimenting with different styles to try to make your

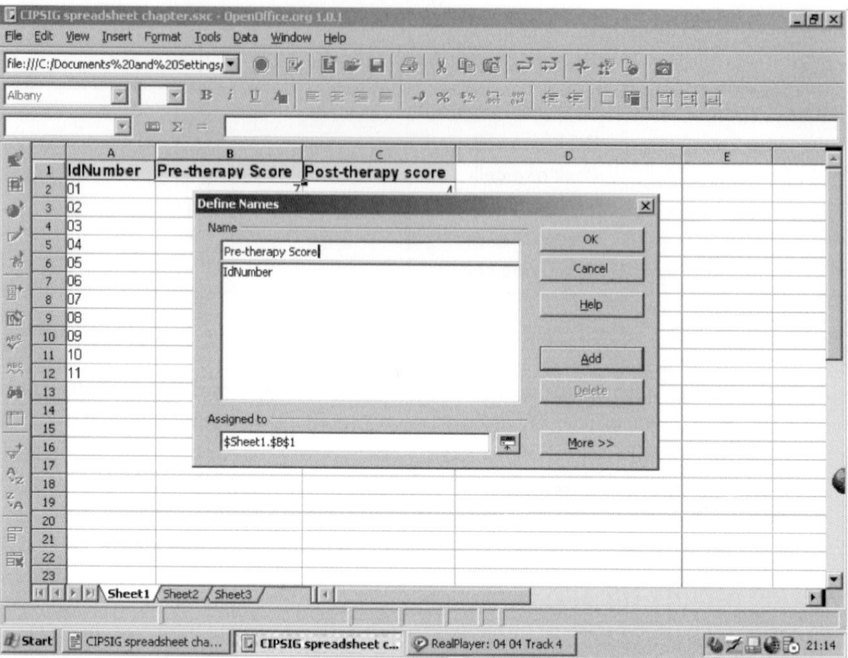

Fig. 5.2 Renaming the first of the default sheets.

spreadsheet easier to read. Figure 5.2, for example, clearly shows the difference between column names and data by putting the former in bold text and putting a different background on those cells.

Resizing cells

To make a row or column larger or smaller, for example when you have a label too big to fit the default cell size, simply click on the edge of the cell and drag the cell border to the correct size. Alternatively, double click on the far cell boundary (the right-hand side for columns and the bottom for rows) and OpenOffice will automatically resize the cell to fit the contents.

Naming columns

The example project used in this chapter (see below) involves three columns: an IdNumber, a pre-therapy score and a post-therapy score. Columns can be named both at the top of the spreadsheet (to make it easy to see which column is which) but also as part of the document. To do this, go to **Insert** → **Names** → **Define** then type in the name of your column in the dialog box (Fig. 5.2). At the bottom of the dialog box is a section titled **Assigned To** and a rather confusing string of characters. If you've never used a spreadsheet package before, these refer to the cells (the boxes you enter data into) that encompass the name of the column. The letters correspond to the columns and the numbers to the rows. Because the clinician has included titles in her spreadsheet, the data for IdNumber would be from A2 (column A, row 2) to A12.

In naming your columns you cannot use spaces or non-alphanumeric characters like – or /. One way around this is to use a mixture of capital and lower-case letters instead, like 'PostTherapyScore' rather than 'Post-therapy Score'.

Entering data

To enter data click on the cell where you wish the data to go and then just type it in. As you type, you'll see exactly the same information being shown in the 'input line' directly above the spreadsheet. This is useful if you want to modify data you have already entered or if you want to type in a complicated formula.

Example of a spreadsheet program in use

The above section gave a very brief and basic overview of using spreadsheets. Here we look at more complicated tasks by using the example of a clinician who wishes to evaluate her clinical work. In this scenario the clinician gives each of her patients a questionnaire at their first appointment and again at the last appointment. Because the sample group is small and the only person to enter and analyse the data is the clinician, she chooses to design a spreadsheet rather than a database. Chapter 6 will expand on this example to look at how evaluative data could be stored at the service-wide level.

The columns used in this spreadsheet are the patient's IdNumber, pre-therapy score and the post-therapy score. The columns are all numerical. Fictitious data have been entered for 11 patients.

Using the spreadsheet

Not just lists

So far the spreadsheet looks just like a list, but there's a lot more you can do to make more sense of the data. You could calculate averages or other equations or create graphs or tables.

To enter formulae, you can click on the **Σ** (sum) button to the left of the input line, or the **Autopilot:Function** button to the immediate left of that.

Calculations

Let's assume you want to calculate the average pre-therapy and post-therapy scores. First, highlight the field you want the calculation to fill (in this case this is in the row two rows below the last record, but the selected field could be anywhere in the datasheet that does not already have data in it). Then click on **Autopilot:Function**. A dialog box appears with a list of possible functions. Select **Average** from the drop-down list and enter the fields to be included in the boxes on the right. You'll see the fields being entered in the Formula section at the bottom of the dialog box. Note that this procedure differs slightly between OpenOffice Calc and Microsoft Excel. In Excel you select the entire range to be included in the calculation rather than specify each individual cell, so averages of pre-therapy scores would be calculated for B2:B12.

There are a huge number of calculations available, including some statistical tests, so experiment with how each works. The potential calculations aren't limited to those in the list either: you can type your own formulae into the cell or input box.

Sorting

You can sort your data to see minimum and maximum values for each column, but take care! Try highlighting column B (or any other column but the first one) and clicking the **Sort Ascending** button. That column sorts from highest to lowest but hasn't changed the order of the other fields. Suddenly our clinician can't match pre- and post-therapy scores to the right patient. To sort fields without this happening, go to **Data** → **Sort**, then select how each column is to be sorted. This way you can sort fields without losing continuity of information.

Filtering

Filtering data involves showing only those records that match criteria set by the user. Our clinician might wish to show only those patients whose questionnaire score fell above a particular level. Clicking on **Data** → **Filter** → **Standard Filter** opens the 'Standard Filter' dialog box. If the cut-off score was 6, she would select *Pre-therapy score* as the field name, >= as the condition, and *6* as the value. Further criteria could be selected to filter by, such as AND (operator) *Post-therapy score* <= *6*. This filter would show all those cases whose pre-therapy questionnaire score was above the cut-off and whose post-therapy score was below the cut-off. This produces five cases. Click on **Data** → **Filter** → **Remove Filter** to show all cases again.

Graphs and charts

Highlight the fields you want to include in the graph. Click on the **Insert Object** button (or **Insert** → **Chart**) to open the **AutoFormat Chart** dialogue box (Fig. 5.3). Here you can designate which cells to include in the graph, specify which cells include row and column labels rather than data,

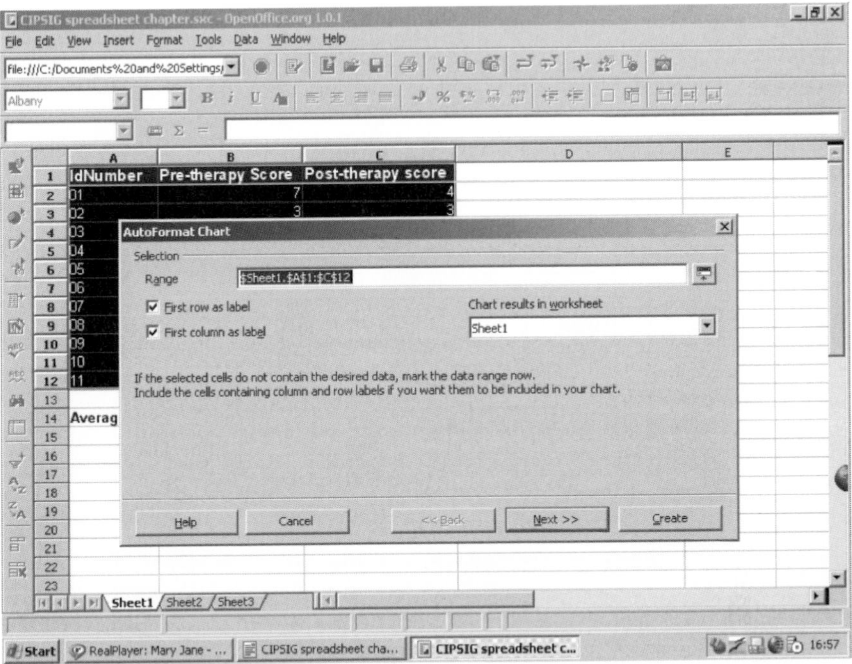

Fig. 5.3 The AutoFormat Chart dialog box.

and select where you want to place the graph in your workbook. For the latter, the default is to insert the graph within the same sheet as the data. While this does allow you to see both the data and the graphs, if you have a lot of data or more than one graph it can look crowded and confused.

Sometimes the data you want for your graph are in non-adjacent cells. In order to create a graph using these columns without moving cells around the data-sheet, highlight one column, then hold down the [CTRL] key and highlight the other. Both columns should now be highlighted but not any in between. Alternatively, you could enter those columns in the **Range** field of the **Autoformat Chart** dialogue box.

For basic data like those used in this example, the choice of graphs is limited. However, if you were to add a few more variables or perform some calculations, the options would be much greater. A more sophisticated graph could be created if you calculate the difference between pre- and post-therapy scores; such a bar graph is shown in Fig. 5,4. This graph shows whether a patient improved or deteriorated between the first and last appointment. Of course, it isn't enough to show why improvements or deteriorations occurred, but that is certainly beyond the scope of this chapter! This graph was created in sheet 2 of the workbook so that it could be enlarged and viewed easily without cluttering up the original data-sheet.

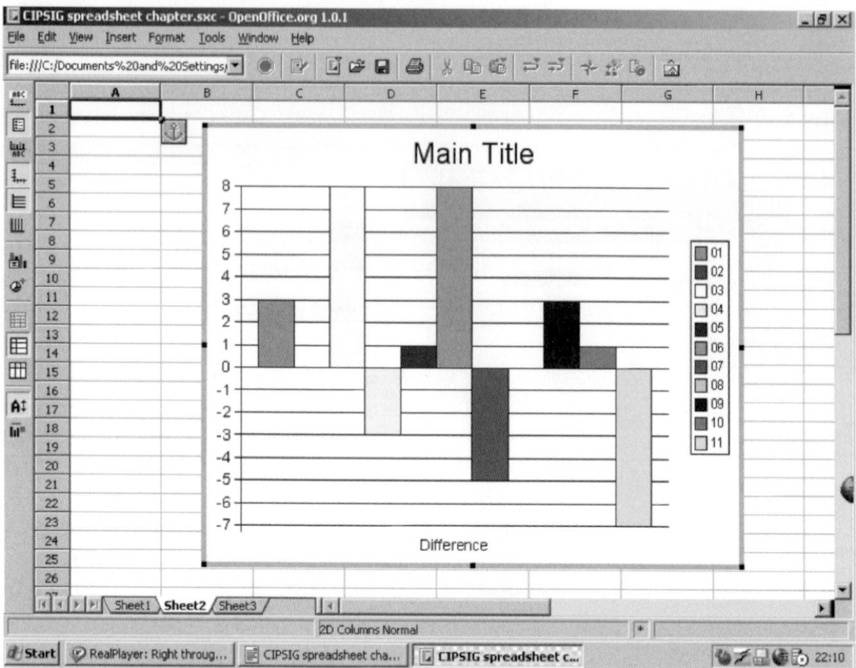

Fig. 5.4 Bar graph of the differences between pre- and post-therapy questionnaire scores.

Standard graphs available in Calc include:

- Column – the default bar chart. This can be used to display almost anything but is particularly useful when you want to compare different populations on the same variable, such as pre-therapy and follow-up questionnaires, waiting times for different projects, or numbers of presenting problems.
- Bar – very similar to column graphs but rotated 90°.
- Line – plots data points linked with a line. This can be used for plotting changes over time, such as problem severity at each appointment.
- Pie – shows how values of a field contribute to the total field. This can be used for analyses like comparing percentages of ethnic categories in a service, or numbers of therapeutic orientations within a clinic.
- Scatter plot – compares pairs of values on *x*- and *y*-axes. This is used for continuous data (e.g. ages, numbers of appointments or questionnaire scores) rather than categorical data (e.g. gender). A scatter plot can be used for analyses such as waiting times by pre-therapy questionnaire scores, or numbers of clinicians with numbers of presenting problems.
- Area – used to compare the degree of change over time. An area plot can be used, for example, to compare changes in waiting times over a given period (such as every month for a year).

- Doughnut – similar to a pie graph but can use multiple fields, such as presenting problems for different clinicians.
- Stock – also called a high–low graph. The term 'stock graph' is used in both Excel and Calc because it is often used for analysing stock market data. It shows the ranges and descriptive values of different fields. It could be used for such analyses as numbers of appointments for different clinical orientations, or questionnaire scores by presenting problems.
- Bubble – similar to a scatter plot but using a third variable, which determines the size of the bubble. So you could look at waiting times by pre-therapy scores with number of presenting problems as the bubble variable.
- Radar – another type of area graph but with variable axes radiating out from a central point. It compares the values of variables on different categories so that the variable with the highest spread across the radar shows the highest value. It could be used for things like individual patient responses to different questionnaire items.
- Surface – shows the best-fit combinations between two sets of data. It could be used, for example, to examine differences between pre-therapy and follow-up questionnaire scores and therapy duration, or number of re-referrals and amount of multi-agency working.
- Cone, cylinder and pyramid – similar to bar and column graphs but with differently shaped bars. These can be used for the same types of analyses.

There are a variety of more specialised graphs available by clicking on the **Custom Types** tab of the 'chart wizard'. It's worth experimenting with these to see what effects you can create.

Conclusion

This chapter should have given you an insight into how to integrate spreadsheets into your practice. If you want to tackle more complex problems a database might be a more appropriate tool and it is to these that we turn in the next chapter.

CHAPTER 6

Databases

Karen Tingay

This chapter aims to give a general overview of databases and their use in mental health, using as an example a service that evaluates its practice using a Microsoft Access database. It is more about how to *use* Access or similar programs in mental health settings than about database theory or design. The version of Access used is from Office 2000, but only minor differences exist between versions. There is also a section at the end on further reading and other database programs, such as MySQL.

What is a database?

A database is a structured collection of data like a spreadsheet table (see Chapter 5). Such a simple structure with only one table is usually referred to as a 'flat-file' database. This chapter focuses largely on more complex 'relational' databases, in which information is stored in several tables that are then linked (or related) together. One advantage of this approach is that it prevents unnecessary repetition; another is that it increases accuracy, as multiple versions of the same information are not maintained. An example of this involving a medical records system is shown in Fig. 6.1.

Advantages and uses of a database

Chapter 5 gave some examples of the use of a spreadsheet in the context of mental health. While a spreadsheet makes an adequate 'flat-file' database, you can see from Fig. 6.1 that each patient visit would require the re-entry of name, date of birth, address and so on, with the inevitable wasted time and errors. For this and other, more technical reasons the flat-file or spreadsheet model does not 'scale' (i.e. grow) robustly with increasing size and complexity. Relational databases manage this complexity by splitting up the information into separate tables and then linking it together in a

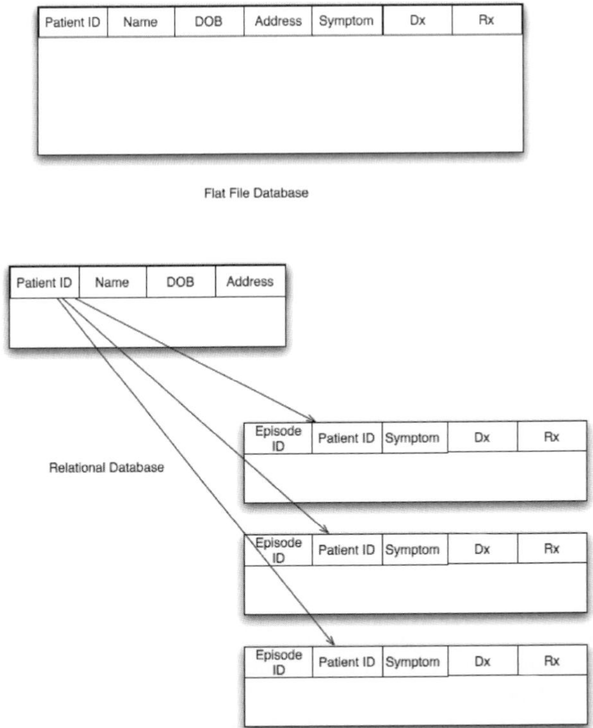

Fig. 6.1 Flat-file and relational database models.

coherent way. It is easier to understand clinical information if it is stored separately from demographic information. The use of relational tables allows the developer to assign codes for fields, which are then used widely throughout the database, such as ethnicity codes as specified by the National Health Service Data Dictionary (2002) or questionnaire codes. These tables can be linked to the main data table.

Thus, many projects that start out using a spreadsheet end up requiring the power that only a database can provide as they grow larger and more complex. On the other hand, tasks that once required a database program, such as address books or reference managers, are now often catered for by specialised software that hides much of the complexity of the underlying database. It is unlikely, however, that the major software companies will release products to manage Care Programme Approach (CPA) lists, or to track community mental health nurses' case-loads, or to allocate resources in a day hospital. Hiring a programmer for one-off tasks like this would be prohibitively expensive, but a tool such as Access allows a non-programmer (albeit a fairly advanced one) to create what are in effect custom applications that hide the gory details of the database behind a user-friendly façade of buttons and screens.

Features of Microsoft Access

Access uses the following tools to enter, store and report on data:

- tables
- queries
- forms
- reports

In addition to these major features we should also mention macros and modules. Macros are little programs that can be used to automate Access. They can be created by recording the actions of the user (see Chapter 3) or by a kind of programming. For example, macros can be created to open up a form that is associated with a particular record based on given criteria, automatically enter data into fields, or to extract data into another format (such as a text file) so that it can be used by other databases. Modules are also used to run routine tasks. They are similar to the web-browser plug-ins discussed in Chapter 10.

Tables

Database tables are very similar to the Calc spreadsheets we looked at in Chapter 5. They are made up of 'records' (rows) and 'variables' or 'factors' (columns), with information being entered in a 'field' (cell) (Fig. 6.2). Tables allow for more choices than do normal spreadsheets, such as the ability to create 'list' and 'combo' (hybrid of text and list) boxes and 'memo' fields. You can also specify detailed criteria for 'correct' entries, such as formats for date fields or upper-case characters. This will be discussed in more detail in the example that follows.

Table relationships

Relationships between tables can be created so that Access 'understands' how data in each table works. A database may have a table containing demographic data on a patient, another containing data on medication, and another containing data on diagnoses or presenting problems. Relationships tell Access that particular medication and diagnostic records refer to a patient.

Queries

These are similar to tables but manipulate data stored in tables to answer questions. Data can be sorted and filtered using varying complexities of criteria; new fields can be calculated from existing data; fields can be updated based on data in other fields, and so on. We will look at some uses for queries in the example below.

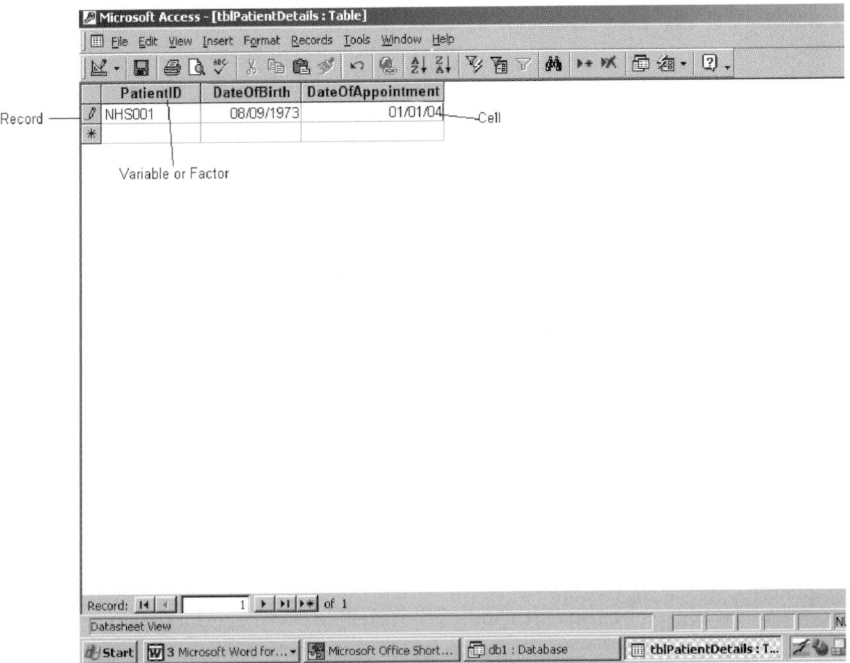

Fig. 6.2 Records, variables and fields in an Access table.

Forms

Forms are the 'front end' or user view of the database. Although data can be entered directly into tables (and rarely into queries), it is more usual and generally easier to create forms. Not only can forms look less confusing than tables, but you can set the form to steer the user in particular ways around the database. For example, if the user enters a particular response (such as 'No' in a yes/no field), the database can then show different fields for more specific data entry than if the user had responded in another way. You can also add buttons or links to other sections of the database to help the user navigate.

Reports

Reports are the parts of the database that are most likely to be printed. They are often built from queries by which the data have been manipulated in some way, for example selecting or grouping certain cases. An example of these types of reports is lists of patients at different stages on waiting lists. In our example we will look at producing reports for an individual patient's questionnaire results, and one on aggregated questionnaire results for an individual clinician's patients.

Example of the use of a database

Let's expand the example in Chapter 5, in which a clinician wanted to evaluate her work by comparing pre-therapy and post-therapy responses to a questionnaire. A spreadsheet may suffice for such a simple task, but if the project were extended to include the rest of the service, a spreadsheet is likely to become too confusing for anyone to use. The overview below should gives you an idea of some of the functions and controls you can include in your forms to make your database easier for users.

To start, open Access and select **Blank Access Database**. Select a suitable name and save the new database to your chosen location in the file system (see Chapter 1). Once saved, Access should bring up the screen shown in Fig. 6.3.

Building tables

To the left of the screen shown in Fig. 6.3 is a list of objects. Clicking on any of the tabs will bring up all the tables, queries, forms and so on that have been created or the means to do so. Access starts in the tables section for new databases or the last modified object for existing databases.

Double click on **Create Table In Design View** (Design View shows the properties of each field in the table, while Datasheet View shows the data

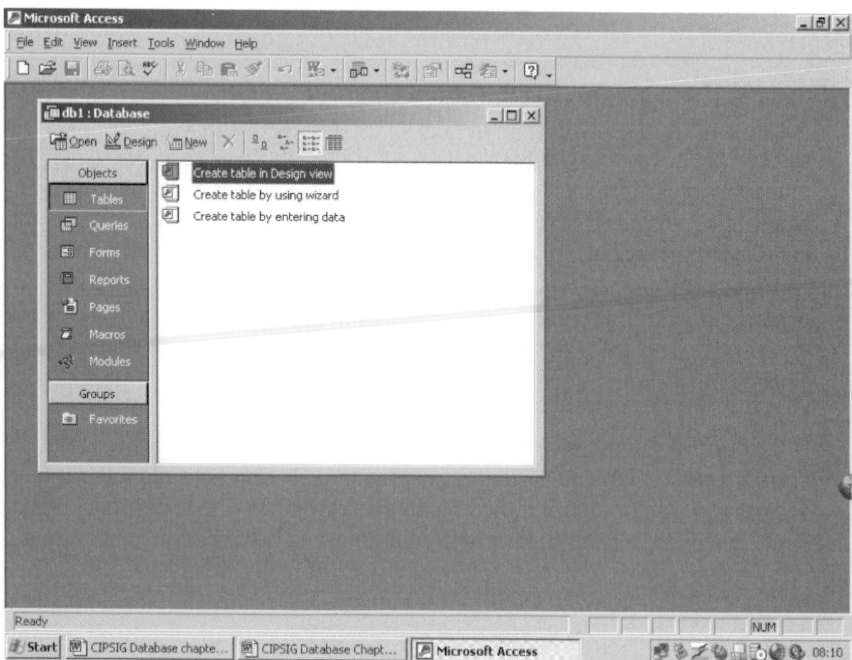

Fig. 6.3 A blank Access database.

within each field). Design View brings up three columns: **Field Name, Data Type** and **Description. Field Name** is self-explanatory, although there are a few conventions to bear in mind. It is best not to use spaces or punctuation marks in your field names and try to keep to the same naming format throughout your database because it makes it easier to remember what your field or table or query or whatever is called without constantly having to check. So if, for example, you've named one field *DateOfBirth*, say, don't name another one *Family_Composition* (and thereby switching from no use to use of the underscore). Picking a good naming format at the beginning can prevent you from spending hours changing all your field names when you realise they are confusing or are causing problems.

The **Data Type** column allows you to determine what type of information, and what information rules, will be used for that field. It is similar to the 'number' categories in Calc and Excel. Most of the data types are self-explanatory but a few need explanation:

- **Autonumber** means Access automatically allocates a sequential number to the field every time a new table row (i.e. a record) is started. These numbers continue sequentially even if you delete a field, so deleting number 30 will still make the next number 31.
- **Hyperlink** makes the value of the field a hyperlink (URL or web address – see Chapter 10).
- **OLE object** refers to pictures, documents, spreadsheets, sounds and so on that can be stored in the database.
- **Memo** allows you to insert long text boxes into your database. For example, you may want to include case notes, letters or clinical reports. Memo fields can be filtered but, unlike text boxes, they can't be sorted.
- **Lookup Wizard** allows you to use data in existing tables, such as ethnicity or gender codes, in another table. We'll go through this in more detail later in this section.

The **Descriptions** column of **Design View** can be useful if you have a large table or tend to use confusing field names like PPreQ for Parent Pre-therapy Questionnaire. Not only is it a reminder to yourself but also to anyone else who might want to modify or fix the database in your place.

Once you've typed in your field name and selected the data type, you'll notice that the **Field Properties** section in the lower half of the screen has changed. Different data types have different properties, so changing will mean modifying the properties too. The main properties to consider are listed in Table 6.1.

In addition, in **Field Properties** you'll see a tab called **Lookup**. This allows you to set the displayed control (as a text box, a list box or a combo box) as well as specifying whether the data options in list boxes or combo boxes come from existing tables or queries. If the displayed control is set to **Text Box** you don't have any other options, but if it's set to **List Box** or **Combo Box** you've got more control over what data are entered. Text

Table 6.1 Table field properties

Field title	Description
Format	For numerical types of data, like number and currency
Input Mask	Allows you to set criteria for 'acceptable' data and to reject any attempts to enter incorrect data, such as mistyped postcodes or dates of birth in a particular numerical sequence like ccyymmdd, for example
Field Size	Used for text and number fields. If you know the data in this field are going to be long, like journal titles or hospital names, set this field accordingly. Smaller fields, however, hold less memory and the table may run faster, so don't set the field size much higher than you're likely to need
Default Value	Handy if you've got a field that's more likely to contain one value than another
Validation Rule	This allows you to set further data entry criteria. For example, if your service sees patients only of a particular age range, you could set the 'AgeAtReferral' field's validation rule to bring up an error message (as set in the Validation Text field below Validation Rule) if the patient's age is entered as anything other than in that range
Required	Whether or not the field requires an entry. If an important field is often left blank you could set this so that anyone entering data wouldn't be able to leave the record without entering something in the field
Indexed	Indexes are used if a field is regularly sorted or grouped. For example, you might want to index a 'Surname' field if your database regularly needs to sort patients by their surname. It helps speed these functions up

boxes are useful if you can't limit what data are going to be entered, such as first name or surname. List and combo boxes are used if you have a limited number of options, such as gender. List and combo boxes are also more useful than text boxes if you later want to look at subsets of data, such as only patients of Asian descent. By setting field value options in this way you can be sure you are not missing records because of typing errors or differing values ('Asian – Indian' isn't the same to Access as 'Asian', for example).

Primary keys

A primary key is set to a field (fields) that contains data unique to a record. It allows all the other items of data for that record to be identified so that if you sort the data they do not become jumbled (as they would in Calc or Excel). A primary key can also act as a 'foreign key', that is, the linking field between two tables. A field containing National Health Service numbers could be set as a primary key, or the combination of first name, surname and date of birth. Primary key fields usually can't contain duplicated information – so you won't enter the same number in different records.

Enter the fields set out in Table 6.2 in your blank table. Set *IdNumber* as the primary key (**Edit → Primary Key**), then save the table as *tblPatientDetails* (**File → Save As**). If you now view the data (**View → Datasheet**) you will see that the patient's IdNumber is automatically entered because this field is an autonumber.

Table 6.2 Fields for tblPatientDetails

Field name	Data type	Description
IdNumber	Autonumber	The patient's identifier
DOB	Date/Time	The patient's date of birth
GenderID	Number	The patient's gender

Look-up tables

In a new table (in Design View) create the fields set out in Table 6.3. Set *GenderID* as the primary key and save the table as *tblGenderCodes*. (I find that naming database objects using a prefix like tbl, qry, frm or rpt avoids confusion if you have similar names for each.) In Datasheet View type in the values shown in Table 6.4 (taken from the National Health Service Data Dictionary 'Sex' codes, 2004).

In Design View of *tblPatientDetails* click on *GenderID* and set its data type as **Lookup Wizard**. Follow the instructions, taking values from *tblGenderCodes* and using both *GenderID* and *Gender* in the fields to take data from, then save *tblPatientDetails*. Under the **Lookup** tab for ***GenderID*** in *tblPatientDetails* you'll now see that the row source has changed to:

```
SELECT[tblGenderCodes].[GenderID],[tblGenderCodes].[Gender]
FROM tblGenderCodes
```

This is an example of Structured Query Language or SQL, which many databases use. What the example above means is that the data options in this combo box come from the *GenderID* and *Gender* fields of *tblGenderCodes*. If you open *tblPatientDetails* in Datasheet View and click in the Gender field, you should now see the same list of possible codes as those entered in *tblGenderCodes*.

Table 6.3 Fields for tblGenderCodes

Field Name	Data Type
GenderID	Number
Gender	Text

Table 6.4 Gender codes

GenderID	Gender
0	Not specified
1	Male
2	Female
9	Not known

Now go to **Tools** → **Relationships**. You should see both *tblPatientDetails* and *tblGenderCodes* with a line running between them. This line shows that the two tables hold related data, in this case gender codes. These relationships should be created automatically, but if this is not the case, or you want to create a new relationship, highlight the field from the first table in the **Relationship** screen and drag and drop it over the field in the related table. A dialogue box will ask you to confirm the fields linking the two tables.

Other relationships between tables could occur if related information is stored in more than one table. A database may have a table for demographic details, another for clinical details and another for an evaluation questionnaire. Each of these tables would have a common field or fields such as the patient's identification number, that would, in effect, tie the tables together.

Building queries

Once you have some data in your table(s) you might want to start examining them in more detail. Queries are an excellent way to do this.

There are several different types of query.

Select queries

These are probably the most common. In these you filter, sort or calculate fields based on whatever criteria you choose. Therefore, you might build a select query to show how many diagnoses of attention-deficit hyperactivity disorder a clinician made over the past year, or to calculate average ages for a clinical project. Routine calculations such as counting, averages, standard deviations, maximum or minimum values or 'where' statements (i.e. the query should select only those fields where the stated criteria have been met) can be performed on fields by using the **Totals** command. Less routine calculations can be entered manually into the query field.

Select queries make good data-cleaning tools because you can create a query to highlight regular data-entry or report errors that may then be fixed using update queries.

Update queries

These allow you automatically to enter data in one table based on data in the same or another table. For example, you could create an update query to enter a value of 'Not returned' for patients for whom follow-up questionnaires were sent out over a month ago (using the criteria that questionnaires were sent on a date more than a month before the date you are running the query and which haven't yet been returned). Alternatively, you could assume that any patient last seen over a year ago is likely to have stopped coming to the clinic and update a closure field to 'Closed'.

It's a good idea to check your results in Datasheet View before running an update query because the changes are irreversible.

Crosstab queries

These permit the grouping of data such as prevalence of a presenting problem according to patient gender or age ranges of patients seen by different clinicians. One field represents the crosstab rows and another the columns; and then one field (or a calculation of a field) represents the crosstab value. Additional fields can narrow the query further by providing more stringent selection criteria.

Append queries

These are useful if you regularly have to add additional data from other tables, such as aggregating data from databases held at different sites. As with update queries, you should always check your results in Datasheet View before running the query as, once run, this cannot be undone. It might also be sensible to back up your database before doing this.

Make Table queries

These do exactly what the name suggests. You can create a new table from fields and data in existing tables. I have seen these used to help create clinical reports when the existing tables and data are not set up in such a way as to make these reports work.

Delete queries

These are used to delete large chunks of data matching particular criteria, such as obvious data errors that can't be fixed any other way.

Creating a Select query

Click on **Insert → Query → Design View**, then select the table(s) and/or query(ies) whose data you want to examine. You can have quite a few different tables or queries forming part of your new query, but the more tables or queries there are, the slower the query will run. You may also find that your new query may be too complicated. In that case consider crafting a less ambitious one or starting off with smaller queries and then using these to build more detailed ones.

Bear in mind that any tables or queries you select must either have or be capable of having a data relationship: you can't try to build a query using unrelated data stores or your computer will sulk and the query will have very odd results if it works at all. If you haven't already created relationships between your chosen tables or queries, you can do so in the Query Builder window (the Design View where you build your query) by dragging and dropping the appropriate fields from one table/query into another.

The top part of the Query Builder window shows all the tables or queries you're using and all relationships that exist between them. The bottom part of the window is where you tell Access what fields to look at and using what criteria. The Fields row contains the field names. You can use existing fields or create new ones. The Table row states the location of the field being referred to (either directly in the case of existing fields or indirectly in the case of new fields) in the Field row. The Sort row specifies which fields will be sorted and in what order. The default is the first field selected or the primary key field. The **Show** check box allows you to hide fields you don't want shown in the query results. The Criteria rows allow you to set your selection criteria. You can add as many criteria as you want by going to **Insert → Rows**. Criteria can be in any format used in table fields, such as 'Mother', <10 or >#01/01/01# (date values are always surrounded by hashes in queries). 'Wildcards' are symbols that denote variations in the values being selected. For example, an asterisk is used to denote any character: thus Clin* would bring up any field value starting with 'Clin', such as 'Clinician', 'Clinical' and 'Clinically'. A wildcard placed before the value would look for the value in any position in the field other than at the beginning of the field.

Then just drag and drop the fields you're interested in into the Field row in the lower half of the screen and set your query.

Interactive queries

You can create a query that prompts the user for the criteria to be used to select particular cases. This means that you can have one query perform different functions rather than build several almost identical queries. In the Criteria row of the desired field, enter a prompt and enclose it in square brackets. For example:

Like [Please choose a value] & "*"

When run, the query will bring up a parameter box first, asking which value to display. The query will then run using the value entered by the user. The text in square brackets is the parameter question, the wildcard in quotes above tells Access to search for whatever is typed into the parameter box. Again, this type of query will look for values at the start of the field. To look for values anywhere in the field use something like this:

Like "*" & [Please choose a value] & "*"

Building forms

Select **Insert → New Form** then select *tblPatientDetails* (the table containing the data the form will be built from) from the drop-down list at the bottom. You should find yourself in a screen similar to the one shown in Fig. 6.4. The grey area is the 'Form detail'. This can be modified (e.g. in size or colour) by clicking on the **Properties** command button.

Highlight all three fields ([SHIFT] + click) and drag them across to the form detail area. The position of these fields can be modified by dragging them to the correct spot. The toolbox contains various other objects you may want to include in your form. All of these can easily be inserted into your form using an automatic wizard. For example, check boxes are used

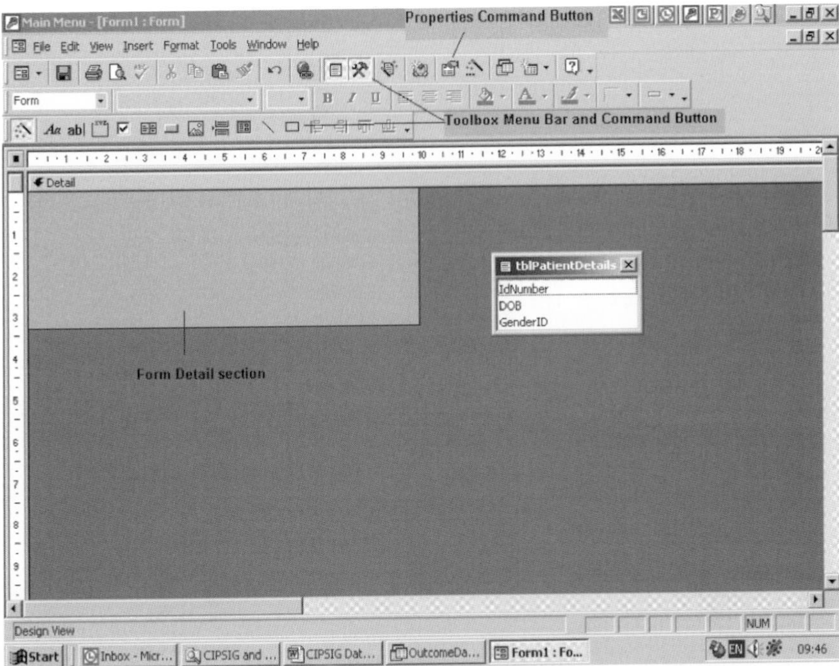

Fig. 6.4 A blank form.

with yes/no fields. Option groups are used in a similar way to check boxes but can include more than one option. For example, you might create an option group for a questionnaire with three possible responses: Not true, Somewhat true and Certainly true. You can select only one response for each option group. List boxes and combo boxes are pretty much the same thing, in that both contain lists of field values. List boxes show all values at the same time, while combo boxes are drop-down lists that you view by clicking on the arrow on the right-hand side of the box.

Command buttons allow you to perform routine tasks by clicking on an easily definable section of the form. For example, you might create a command button to close the form the user is currently in, take the user to a new record, save the existing record, open a report, or even calculate the value of a field based on other field values, even if those other fields are in different forms (as long as all the forms required are open). The **SDQ Score Sheet** command button in Fig. 6.5, for example, opens a new database which is used for scoring the particular questionnaire. It's easiest to use the command button wizard to create these. This should start automatically when you click on the command button section of the toolbox.

Tab controls will create different 'pages' within your form. You may, for example, have different tabs for pre- and post-therapy questionnaires, or to separate demographic, referral, clinical and non-clinical data. Using tabs means the user doesn't constantly have to move between different forms.

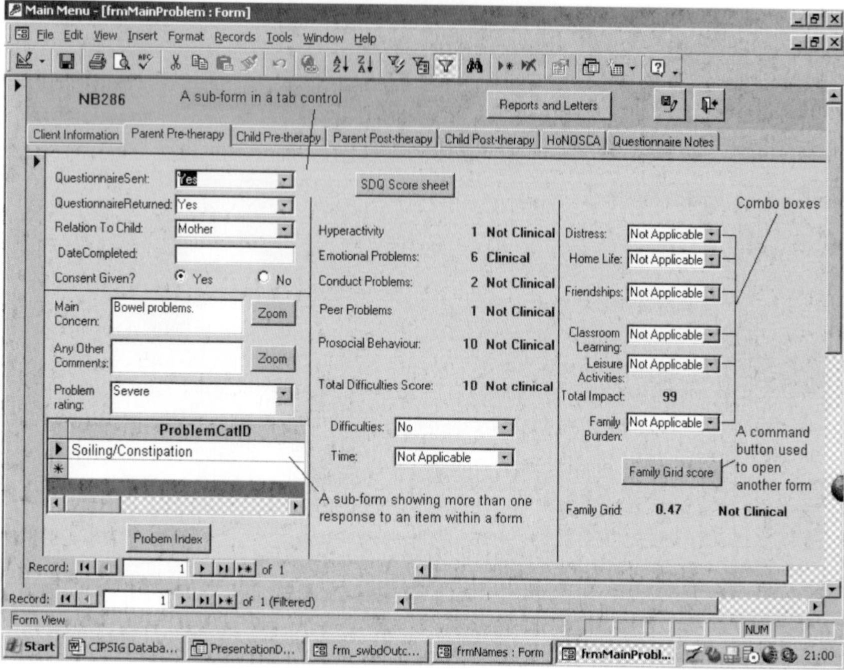

Fig. 6.5 Controls used in a form.

Sub-forms are existing forms inserted into other forms. Sub-forms could be used with tab controls so that a main form would consist of numerous sub-forms, reached by clicking on the tabs. Or they may be instances in which more than one response, such as a presenting problem, clinician or clinical intervention, is relevant to a single episode, such as an assessment or care spell. Figure 6.5 shows how sub-forms, command buttons, tab controls, option groups (the 'Consent Given' field) and combo boxes could work in a clinical database.

Other tools are available using the ActiveX controls found in the **Insert** menu. These include the option to use music and videos, web search engine fields, and email, among others. Some ActiveX controls may require non-standard parts of Access to be installed.

Reports

Reports are another way of making data more comprehensible to users. Information is selected and displayed according to the nature of the report but is usually intended to be printed for more permanent records. Because of this, most reports are created from queries rather than tables. Reports could be created for waiting times, to display patient aggregates for an individual clinician, or even for individual patient information.

Reports are built using similar methods to forms only without such scope to interact with the data once the report has been opened. But all the controls found in forms, such as option groups, can be used in reports.

There is also the ability to group sets of data according to user-defined specifications. For example, a clinician could produce a report looking at patients grouped by age, then presenting problem, then outcome. Or a service-level report could be produced looking at the duration of therapy of patients seen by different clinical teams, further broken down by individual clinicians within those teams.

Using graphs in reports is a very simple and space-saving way of displaying information. A report could be created solely as a graph report (**Insert → Report → Chart Wizard**) or by embedding graphs with other controls, such as tables. In this way a service could design reports showing demographic, referral and clinical data for an individual patient, with graphs for outcome data.

Further reading

Unfortunately there isn't the space in this chapter to look at all the tools Access contains but the further reading list below may help. Also listed are databases other than Access. There are very few books available on using databases in health settings, but most of the examples can be modified or adapted to suit. (Visit the Access section of the Microsoft Office website for tricks, tips, articles and discussions. Some of this can get pretty technical. See *http://office.microsoft.com/en-us/FX010857911033.aspx*).

Anderson, V. (1999) *Access 2000: The Complete Reference*. Berkeley, CA: Osborne/McGraw-Hill.

Callahan, E. (1997) *Microsoft Access 97/Visual Basic. Step by Step*. Washington, DC: Microsoft Press.

Callahan, E. (1999) *Microsoft Access 2000/Visual Basic for Applications. Fundamentals*. Washington, DC: Microsoft Press.

Kaulfeld, J. (1999) *Access 2000 for Windows for Dummies*. Hoboken, NJ: Wiley Press.

Prague, C. N. & Irwin, M. R. (1999) *Access 2000 Bible*. New York: Hungry Minds Inc.

Non-Access databases

Allen, S. & Terry, E. (2005) *Beginning Relational Data Modeling*. Berkeley, CA: Apress.

Elmasri, R. & Navathe, S. B. (1994) *Fundamentals of Database Systems*. Redwood City, CA: Benjamin/Cummings Publishing.

Powell, T. A. (2002) *Web Design: The Complete Reference*. Berkeley, CA: Osborne/McGraw-Hill. (Although not a database book, this describes the principles of screen design.)

Quin, L. (2000) *Open Source XML Database Toolkit*. New York: John Wiley & Sons.

Sheldon, R. & Moes, G. (2005) *Beginning MySQL*. Indianapolis, IN: Wiley Publishing.

Welling, L. & Thomson, L. (2001) *PHP and MySQL Web Development*. Indianapolis, IN: SAMS Publishing.

CHAPTER 7

Research, computers and statistics programs

Stuart Leask

An idiot's guide to research

Research is fun. If you've ever felt certain that a simple question *must* have a simple answer, you are a potential researcher (however wrong you may be in thinking this). Research involves thinking up interesting questions that can be answered. You may want to ask 'How can I make my patients well?' As formulated, this question is too vague to be useful. However, if you become more specific, say what you're proposing to *do* and how you're going to measure the effect, then the question becomes answerable. For example, 'If a patient takes 20 mg of this tablet daily for 6 weeks, does the Beck Depression Inventory score fall by more than the score of a patient taking 20 mg of another tablet, on average?'

Theses and hypotheses

A thesis is a general belief, such as 'The sun rises every morning', which one can argue for and against by means of competing hypotheses, such as 'Every morning it gets light all over the place'. A common hypothesis is the null hypothesis – 'There is no difference in these two (or more) groups'. Alternatively, one may have a more specific hypothesis, a 'research hypothesis' (such as the one above). The hypothesis is a statement; for it to be a scientific hypothesis, it needs to be *demonstrably* true or false – that is, it has to be 'testable'.

To do a study you *must* have a hypothesis. So make sure you have one, and can tell people what it is.

Statistics

I will say more about statistics later, but please, *please* get some statistical advice *at the point of formulating your hypothesis*. There no point in doing a study that has no chance of generating statistically convincing results – no one will ever believe your thesis if the statistics say the results you have could very likely be the result of pure chance. Talk to a colleague with some experience in this area early on to avoid wasting your life.

Sampling

If you just want to answer the question in your own patients, test the hypothesis in your own patients, and don't worry about sampling. However, you may want your findings to be more generally applicable to other people's patients, or even the general population. To make this more likely, you must think about the process that will extract the people you're going to test your hypothesis on from the more general population to which you want your results to generalise. Sampling biases can be insidious and unobvious, so seek advice.

Control groups and placebos

An important comparison with any intervention is what happens if you do nothing. For example, some conditions resolve spontaneously. A common solution is to recruit a group of 'control' patients, for whom nothing special is done, and compare the study group with them. In a treatment trial, the controls may be given the 'normal' treatment or a placebo.

Confounding

You may hope that any differences between the groups you're looking at are arising only because of the difference you are investigating. However, there may be other, 'confounding' explanations. For example, a case–control study confirms that having a box of matches in your pocket increases your risk of developing lung cancer, but your thesis that carcinogenic phosphorous in matches is absorbed through the trousers might be confounded by the association between carrying matches and smoking!

Ethics

Another complication is that we can't experiment upon our patients as if they were guinea pigs. Whatever happens to them must be ethically justifiable. Thus, one often has to compare a new treatment with so-called 'active placebos' or 'conventional treatment', rather than with nothing. You will nearly always need to submit your proposed study protocol to a local research ethics committee (LREC), which will consider whether your study is worth doing, taking into account the risks proposed to the patients and the likelihood (in their view) that you are going to learn anything useful from it. Learn from this process!

Significance versus effect size

Let us say that your new treatment cures 0.1% more patients than the old (the 'effect size'). Even if this is highly significant (that is, terribly unlikely to have happened by chance), it may be that no one will care about such a tiny improvement. The result may be *statistically* significant, but with a small effect size have little *clinical* significance.

On the other hand, another study may determine that a new treatment cures 300% more patients than the old one, what would be called a large effect size, and of course this would be of great interest to clinicians. However, sometimes even such results can arise by chance (perhaps you treated only four patients, and they were lucky), and the result would not be 'statistically significant'.

Both descriptions – effect size and significance – are important. Clearly, you want a result that is significant both statistically *and* clinically.

Measuring instruments

However you divide your participants (cases/controls, active treatment/placebo, etc.), you will need to measure the outcome of interest. The measurement must be valid and reliable, that is, it should be measuring what you say it's measuring, and it should give the same result in a given patient regardless of who is using it. The usual solution is to use a measuring instrument that someone else has already used and shown to be valid and reliable. Another advantage is that there will be some normative data on the tool's performance, which is very useful for the 'power calculation' (see below). If you are inventing your own tool, you'll need to validate it and demonstrate its reliability, a process beyond the scope of this brief chapter.

Masking (blinding)

The reason why drug trials are often 'masked' or 'blinded' (i.e. participants don't know if they are taking the active drug or placebo) is that a doctor's or a patient's expectations can confound a trial outcome. For example, patients may modify their symptoms, and a doctor may modify how they interpret these, depending on whether or not they think an active treatment is being prescribed. If you are recording something from patients' case notes, you may be biased if you see they have a particular diagnosis.

Power calculations

Whatever you're investigating, it is important to have some idea that your study has a chance of getting a statistically significant result; this is the only way of convincing others. If you're trying a new treatment in a field where nothing works, an initial study may need only a few cases to demonstrate that this treatment works. However, in the real world, current treatments often do work, and patients can spontaneously remit, so you may need quite a few successes to demonstrate that a new treatment is significantly better than the old.

A power calculation takes into account how much spread you're going to get in the results in each group, and how different you're expecting the groups to be. It then calculates how many participants you're going to need in your study to have a good chance of getting a statistically significant result. If there is a lot of spread with your measuring instrument, or if the differences you're looking for are small, you'll need many participants. If the spread is small and/or the differences you're expecting are big, you'll need fewer.

Recording your data

Writing your data down is a good idea. Computer spreadsheets are useful for storing tabulated data (see Chapter 5), but they occasionally crash and lose data, and you might dutifully enter this week's data in the wrong column; either way, a paper 'original' will give you something to check later. A paper record can also support patient anonymity; allocate a 'study ID' to each patient, record data on sheets with only the ID, and keep the list relating names to IDs separately, under lock and key. This will soothe your local ethics committee no end. There are computer packages (e.g. the free program Epi Info™) that enable you to design electronic response forms which can overcome many of these issues, but these are beyond the scope of this chapter.

Consider that how you record data should reflect how you're going to analyse them – record only the information you are going to use. Recording data as precisely as possible is wise; for example, if you're comparing 'tall' and 'short' people, record their height and worry about the cut-off later.

Try out your 'data recording forms' *before* you start for real. You'll often discover that there's not enough space for 'this', more space than you'll ever need for 'that' and nowhere to write 'the other'. If someone else is to use them, are they filled in correctly? Have some questions been misinterpreted? 'Pilot' your measures with a few people to check this side of things, rather than getting back 5000 forms all filled in wrongly! This way you can change the form before it's too late. Don't forget, 'garbage in = garbage out': if the data are recorded wrongly or ambiguously, no amount of clever analysis will correct your findings.

Eyeballing your data

Once you have some data, you need to analyse them. *You* need to look at the recorded results. Do they make sense? Are they what you expected? Are they consistent? Did the forms get filled in wrongly (despite your efforts earlier)? Were they accurately transcribed to your computer database? Even nonsensical data can be used to generate test statistics. You need to feel happy you can defend the reliability and validity of your raw data.

Descriptive statistics

Once you have your results, you will want to summarise them. If they are normally distributed, a mean and standard deviation may be appropriate. If they are categorical, tables of counts and percentages are a start. Ideally, your initial hypothesis will have been formulated specifically enough for it to tell you what summaries you want, say, 'The patients in group A will have a lower mean serum plutonium level than those in group B'.

Statistical tests

Broadly speaking, for simple studies you will usually want to compare either two continuous measures (e.g. two serum levels or scale scores) or two categorical measures (e.g. numbers of patients). What emerges from this is a figure that expresses the likelihood (1 = certain, 0 = impossible) that the result you have could be the result of chance. This is the magical '*P* value'.

For a research hypothesis, $P < 0.05$ means that there is a less than 0.05 (5%) probability that your findings are just the result of random chance. For a null hypothesis $P < 0.05$ means that there is a less than 5% probability that this result is actually the same as no change. To put it another way, $P = 0.05$ means that if you did the study 20 times, you would fail to demonstrate your finding only once. The bottom line is that most people will accept that yours is a real finding if *P* is less than 0.05.

Data presentation

'A picture paints a thousand words' – consider how you want to present your findings. Tables of numbers, although dull, are better than using pretty graphs that don't add anything. Histograms show how results are distributed, bar charts compare counts or proportions, and line graphs show relationships (e.g. between two variables, or changes over time).

Try to present data once only – if that's in a table, don't replicate those results in a graph without good reason. Remember that even the prettiest graph that isn't easy to appreciate, or just duplicates data shown elsewhere, will only irritate a busy reader. Effective data presentation is about effective communication, so reviewing the chapters in this book on word processing and presentations can also help you get this right (see Chapters 3 and 4).

Umm … thinking …

Working out exactly what you've done, what you've found and what it means will take *time*. It is not uncommon to find that the thinking process takes longer than the data-gathering process. Allow plenty of time to do this – weeks or even months: don't assume you'll be able to work it all out in a few days.

Finally

Write up why you thought anyone would be interested in doing what you did, what you did and how you did it, what you found and whether the results were statistically significant. Then briefly discuss your findings, how these differ from previous work and (perhaps) why, what the consequences might be for clinicians and policy-makers, what important questions remain and what work might sensibly follow.

Then pop it in an envelope to the *Lancet*: glory awaits!

Statistics software

Most statistics packages can perform the basic analyses required for simple studies. Packages such as SPSS can perform all but the most abstruse of analyses, although these abilities come at a price: a licence for SPSS can cost thousands of pounds.

At various points in this book, we have highlighted the existence of free software alternatives (free in terms of both cost and draconian licensing conditions). We'll show you how to use the R statistical package, as it is free to download and therefore available to readers regardless of their financial or professional status. Widely used in the physical sciences, R is also very well suited to medical research statistics. Informal support is available by means of websites, as well as an enthusiastically supported 'Help' list. R is available for many computing platforms; the text below describes the Microsoft Windows version, but users of other operating systems (Macintosh, Linux, etc.) should find things similar once the program is installed. Explanations will also cater for users of SPSS.

Obtaining R

To ensure you get the very latest version of R go to *http://www.r-project.org/* and follow the 'download' links. Make sure you download the relevant version for your operating system. See the material on downloading and installing programs in Chapter 1.

Make sure to save the program somewhere you can find it again (the desktop is good). Run the R install program (the icon looks like a little PC with a CD) by double clicking on it. It's OK to accept the options the installation program gives you. You will now have a big R icon (a 'shortcut') on your desktop.

Start R by double clicking on the big R icon. You'll get a rather spartan empty window. Real R pros operate by typing commands straight into this window and studying the messages R sends back. For newcomers, there is a graphical user interface (GUI) to help, called R Commander. It takes instructions from you by means of user-friendly menus and types the arcane commands for you.

First, prepare R so it uses multiple windows on your main desktop, rather than multiple sub-windows in its own window. Edit the R shortcut by right clicking on the shortcut and selecting **Properties**. Then add the characters *--sdi* to the end of the text in the **Target** box (Fig. 7.1), so it reads `"C:\Program Files\R\rw2001\bin\Rgui.exe" --sdi`. (If R won't connect to the internet you could try adding a space and `--internet2` after `sdi` at this step).

Next, load R Commander. From the **Packages** menu at the top of the R window, select **Install Package(s) from CRAN**. A long list of add-on packages should appear. Locate and click on **Rcmdr**, and the GUI plus all required libraries will be automatically downloaded and installed.

Now load the R Commander library into the R workspace by typing `library(Rcmdr)` into the R window at the prompt. (Hit return after typing each line in R.) Another window will open, with lots of familiar options to load and save data, and less familiar ones to do analyses and print graphs. Note that R is 'case sensitive' – typing `Rcmdr` is different from `rcmdr` or `RCMDR`. This is useful in the long run, but can catch you out at first. Note, too, that parentheses – curly or square brackets – `library[Rcmdr]` – won't work.

Once R Commander is running, we will be working in both the R window (or 'R console') and the more interesting R Commander window

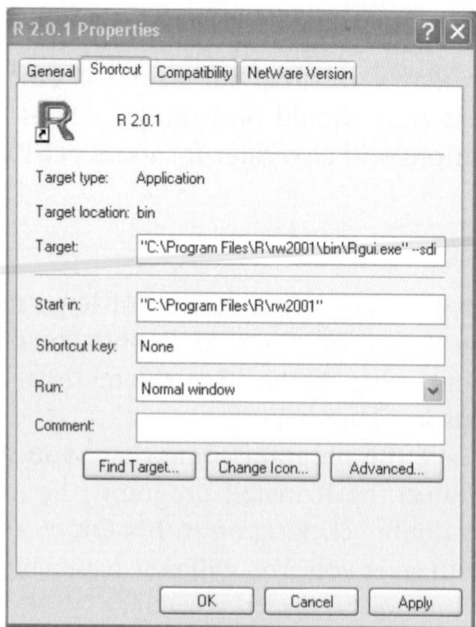

Fig. 7.1 R shortcut properties dialogue box.

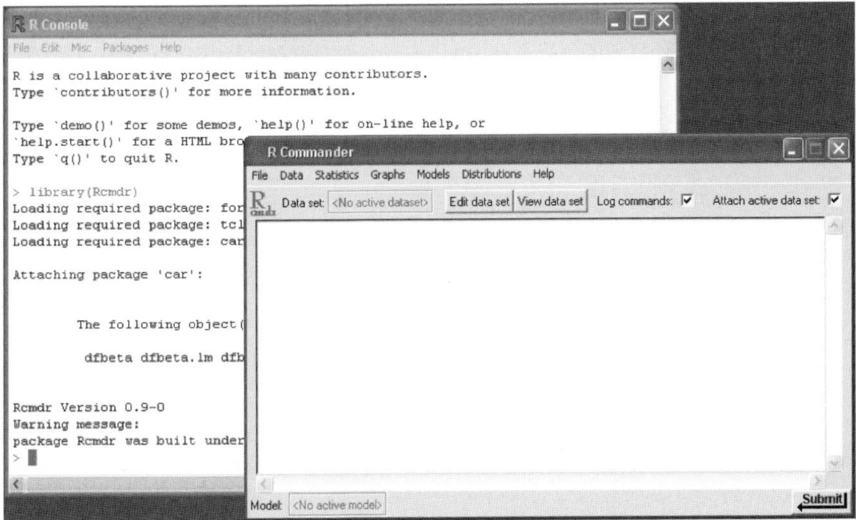

Fig. 7.2 The R console on the left and the R Commander window on the right.

(see Fig. 7.2). If you want to swap between them click on the appropriate rectangle on the taskbar at the bottom of your Windows screen.

We will now use R with its GUI to do the work mentioned in the introductory section: power calculations, entering data, descriptive statistics, basic graphs and statistical tests.

Getting data into R

Getting data into R is easy. Start from the point above, where you're running the R Commander library, and the GUI window is open. In the R Commander window, selecting the option **Data → New Data Set** will open a spreadsheet, with lots of empty boxes for you to put data into, under each variable (var1, var2, var3, etc.) (Fig. 7.3). Try entering some data (any old numbers) for the first three variables. At this stage, keep life simple by making sure there is a number for all three variables for all of the first ten cases (rows). Double clicking on the variable name (e.g. var1) lets you edit the name and the data type (numeric or character) (Fig. 7.4). It is important to set the data type to 'character' for any categorical data you enter. This tells R you consider these as categories in any future analyses – even if the categories are numbers!

When you've finished, close the data editor just as if it were any other program (see Chapter 1).

R does want you to be explicit about whether the data for each variable consists of numbers (1, 2, 1.678, 1003, etc.) or characters (generally words such as Male, Female, Big, Medium, Small, etc.). This is because it

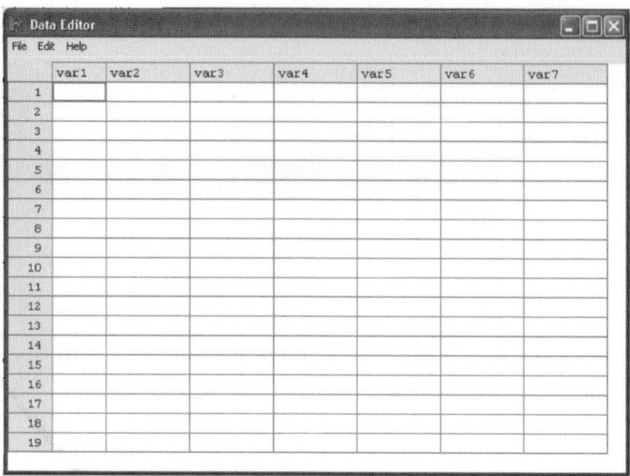

Fig. 7.3 The R data editor.

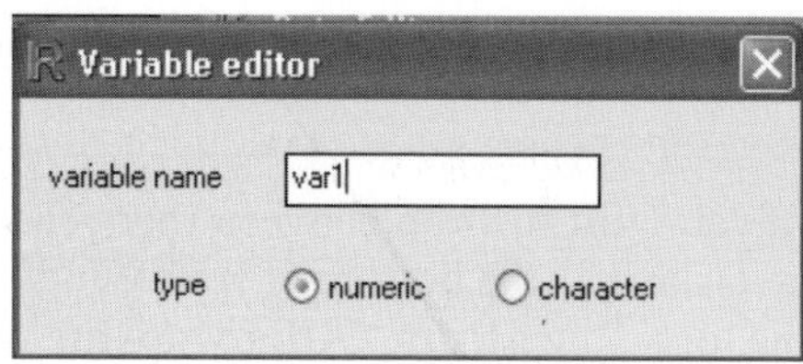

Fig. 7.4 The variable editor.

is immediately obvious what is meant by a number, whereas names can mean anything. In addition, certain analyses are meaningful only with the right sort of data. However, statistical analyses see the world in terms of numbers, so any analysis by gender will just divide your data into two groups anyway. Thus, it is a good discipline to enter your data as numbers from the outset, and make a note of any categorical labelling (e.g. Male = 1, Female = 2) as you go along.

SPSS is similar in this regard: you type data into its spreadsheet. It also offers 'Value labels' if you double click on a variable name at the top of the spreadsheet. A similar facility is available in R.

Once you have finished entering data, you can save from the R Commander **Data** menu (Fig. 7.5): **Data** → **Active data set** → **Export Active Data Set**. You can reload it later using **Data** → **Import Data** → **From Text File**. If you want to edit it, click the **Edit Data** button on the R Commander window (Fig. 7.6).

SPSS offers similar **Save** and **Open** options from the **File** menu, but you can load only one data-set at a time.

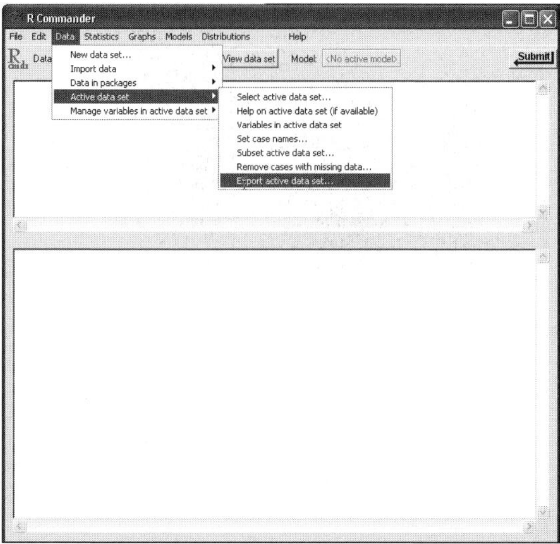

Fig. 7.5 The data-set save menu.

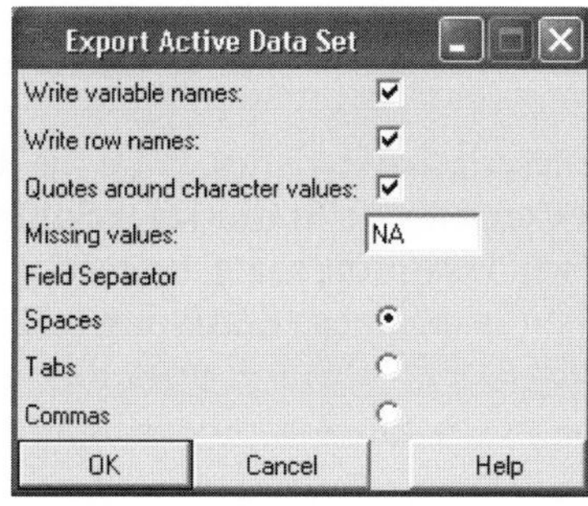

Fig. 7.6 Specifying the data save options.

Assigning names

Although I recommend entering your data as numbers if possible, it is worth being careful what you call your variables too. In R, you can give variables very long names, but you shouldn't use spaces or underscores (_) to make them clearer, as these characters will lead to errors. However, R is case sensitive, so MyVariable as a name would be both readable and unambiguous. Similarly, Gender, SerumRhubarbMMol, IrishStewishness are all unambiguous, informative and readable variable names.

SPSS works with both variable names (but up to a maximum of eight characters) and variable labels (many characters including spaces, often proving very difficult to tabulate). Seasoned SPSS users usually discipline themselves to use brief, meaningful variable names wherever possible.

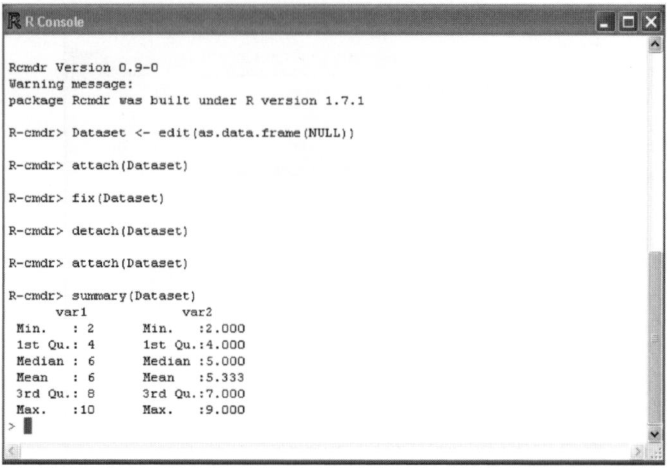

```
R Console

Rcmdr Version 0.9-0
Warning message:
package Rcmdr was built under R version 1.7.1

R-cmdr> Dataset <- edit(as.data.frame(NULL))

R-cmdr> attach(Dataset)

R-cmdr> fix(Dataset)

R-cmdr> detach(Dataset)

R-cmdr> attach(Dataset)

R-cmdr> summary(Dataset)
      var1            var2
 Min.   : 2      Min.   :2.000
 1st Qu.: 4      1st Qu.:4.000
 Median : 6      Median :5.000
 Mean   : 6      Mean   :5.333
 3rd Qu.: 8      3rd Qu.:7.000
 Max.   :10      Max.   :9.000
>
```

Fig. 7.7 Summarising data.

Descriptive statistics

Right, let's do some descriptive statistics. From the R Commander window (as opposed to the R Console), do **Statistics → Summaries → Active Data Set**. The R Console will now print some interesting summaries (Fig. 7.7).

The SPSS equivalent is to choose **Statistics → Descriptives**.

Graphs

Let's make some graphs! Again, from the R Commander menu choose **Graphs → Histogram**, select a variable and click **OK**, *et voilá* – a histogram (Fig. 7.8).

SPSS users can also produce pretty graphs from the **Graph** menu, but R exceeds its commercial rival in flexibility.

R syntax

In R, you can construct the most fiendish of analyses by typing commands straight into the R Console (Fig. 7.9). However, you can see how the R Commander is doing its stuff by looking at the text it is pasting into the R window as you click away with your mouse. As in SPSS, you can save the text of this, and later cut and paste it into the R window. You can add comments to your analyses by using the hash symbol (#) – R will ignore the rest of any line after the hash (see Fig. 7.9). In this way, analyses can be reused or modified.

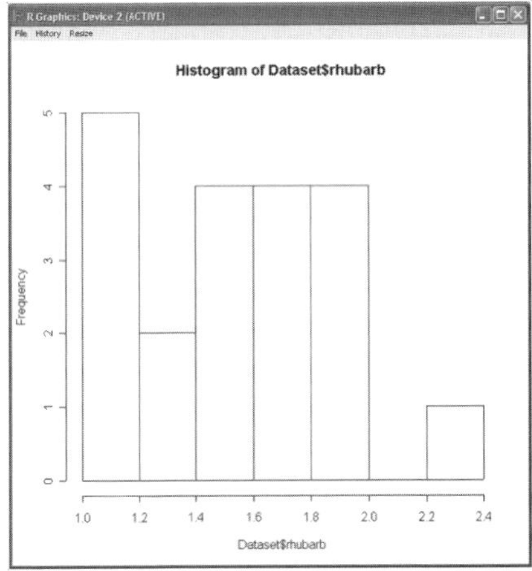

Fig. 7.8 A histogram produced by R.

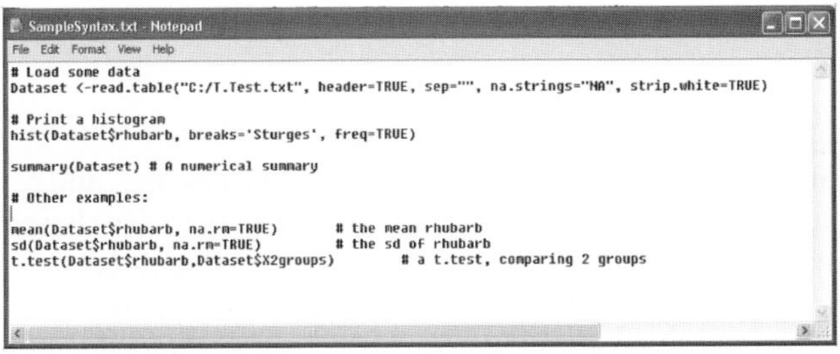

SampleSyntax.txt - Notepad

```
# Load some data
Dataset <-read.table("C:/T.Test.txt", header=TRUE, sep="", na.strings="NA", strip.white=TRUE)

# Print a histogram
hist(Dataset$rhubarb, breaks='Sturges', freq=TRUE)

summary(Dataset) # A numerical summary

# Other examples:

mean(Dataset$rhubarb, na.rm=TRUE)        # the mean rhubarb
sd(Dataset$rhubarb, na.rm=TRUE)          # the sd of rhubarb
t.test(Dataset$rhubarb,Dataset$X2groups)         # a t.test, comparing 2 groups
```

Fig. 7.9 Some R syntax in a text editor.

Power calculations

As mentioned above, power calculations need to be done before you even submit your protocol to the ethics committee. Essentially, you will ask of the power calculation:

'Given what I already know about the performance of my measuring instrument and the difference I am anticipating finding in this study, how many participants will I need to give myself a good likelihood [usually 80%] of demonstrating this result with a high [usually 95%] significance?'

It should be straightforward, for example, to get an idea of the mean and standard deviation of the results of a popular measuring instrument in the population you're interested in. If you have no idea about this, or what sort of difference you may get, a review of the literature in this field may help you get a better idea, especially if it is combined with a small pilot study.

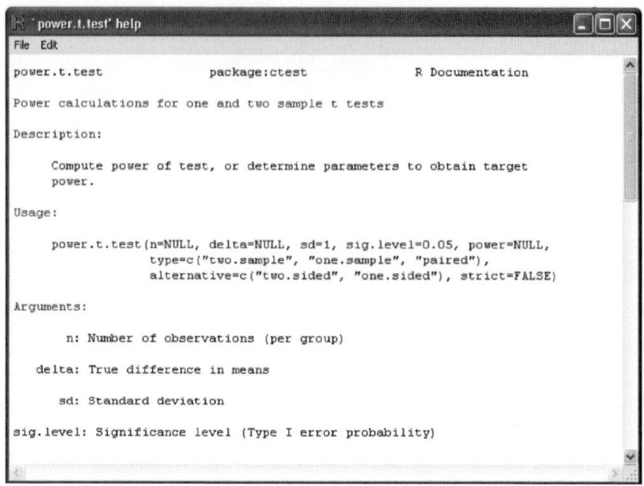

Fig. 7.10 The help pager (for power.t.test).

You then put these figures into a power calculation. In R, you use *power.t.test* for comparing two groups by a continuous measure, and *power.prop.test* to compare counts in two groups. To find out how to use these commands, ask R: type `?power.t.test` into the R console (Fig. 7.10).

Let us assume that, for your first study, you want to know how many participants you'll need to have an 80% chance of spotting a difference of one standard deviation between readings in two groups, with 95% certainty (a significance level of 0.05). Now type this into the R Console:

```
power.t.test(delta=1, sig.level=0.05, power=0.8)
```

As you can see, you'll need just over 16 participants in each group.

Alternatively, you may be looking at proportions. Say you wish to have an 80% chance of spotting that in group 1 50% of cases and in group 2 75% of cases (absolute difference of 25%, from a mean in group 1 of 50%) have the index condition. Figure 7.11 shows the results of the data entry: it looks as if you're going to need 58 cases in each group.

Comparing two groups: t-tests

You can do *t*-tests from R Commander. Load some sample data with **Data → Import Data From Text File**. Load *TTestData.txt* (sample databases available from the book website) in two groups, where group 1 ate no rhubarb whereas group 2 ate lots. After loading *TTestData.txt*, edit the data-set to make sure the grouping variables, groups2 and groups3, are

```
R Console
File Edit Misc Packages Help
You are welcome to redistribute it under certain conditions.
Type 'license()' or 'licence()' for distribution details.

R is a collaborative project with many contributors.
Type 'contributors()' for more information.

Type 'demo()' for some demos, 'help()' for on-line help, or
'help.start()' for a HTML browser interface to help.
Type 'q()' to quit R.

> power.prop.test(p1=.50, p2=.75, power=.80)

     Two-sample comparison of proportions power calculation

              n = 57.67344
             p1 = 0.5
             p2 = 0.75
      sig.level = 0.05
          power = 0.8
    alternative = two.sided

 NOTE: n is number in *each* group

>
```

Fig. 7.11 Power for proportions.

character and not numeric variables. (Note that R can also open SPSS and Minitab data files from R Commander, and other formats (e.g. SAS) using syntax commands.)

Say you wish to see whether the (normally distributed) values of serum rhubarb differ significantly. Using the R Commander menus, go to **Statistics → Means → Independent Samples T-Test**. You then pick your response variable (rhubarb) and your grouping variable (groups2). As you can see in the R window (Fig. 7.12), the *P* value is 0.048, which suggests

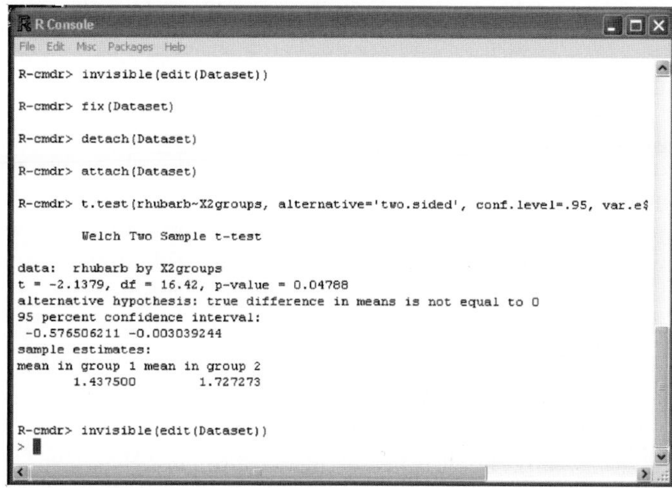

```
R Console
File Edit Misc Packages Help
R-cmdr> invisible(edit(Dataset))

R-cmdr> fix(Dataset)

R-cmdr> detach(Dataset)

R-cmdr> attach(Dataset)

R-cmdr> t.test(rhubarb~X2groups, alternative='two.sided', conf.level=.95, var.e$

        Welch Two Sample t-test

data:  rhubarb by X2groups
t = -2.1379, df = 16.42, p-value = 0.04788
alternative hypothesis: true difference in means is not equal to 0
95 percent confidence interval:
 -0.576506211 -0.003039244
sample estimates:
mean in group 1 mean in group 2
       1.437500        1.727273


R-cmdr> invisible(edit(Dataset))
>
```

Fig. 7.12 Output of a t-test.

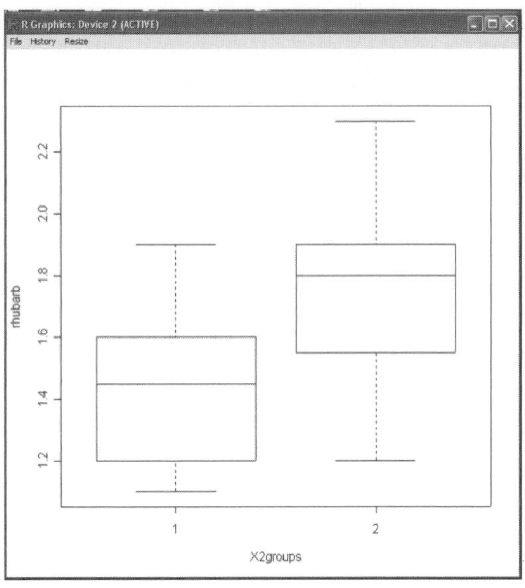

Fig. 7.13 Boxplot.

that there is a less than a 5% probability of getting these group differences by chance. It looks as if eating rhubarb affects your serum rhubarb levels after all.

A boxplot might illustrate the group difference well. Use **Graphs → Boxplot** for the rhubarb variable, then the Plot by groups option to choose the groups2 variable. The result is shown in Fig. 7.13.

Analysis of variance

If you have more than two groups, say a control group, treatment 1 and treatment 2, rather than separately comparing each group against the others (and thus being guilty of so-called 'multiple testing', which can under-estimate your *P* value) it is usually more correct to perform an analysis of variance (ANOVA). In this data-set, to illustrate this point there is another grouping variable called groups3. Use **Statistics → Means → One-way ANOVA** (one-way, as you're looking only at the effect of one factor on the outcome variable). Again, look at serum rhubarb, but group using the variable groups3, which notionally considers that data has come from three groups instead of two. As you can see (Fig. 7.14), the probability of getting this partitioning at random is very low. The boxplot (**Graph → Boxplot** and add the new grouping variable as before) shows the results graphically.

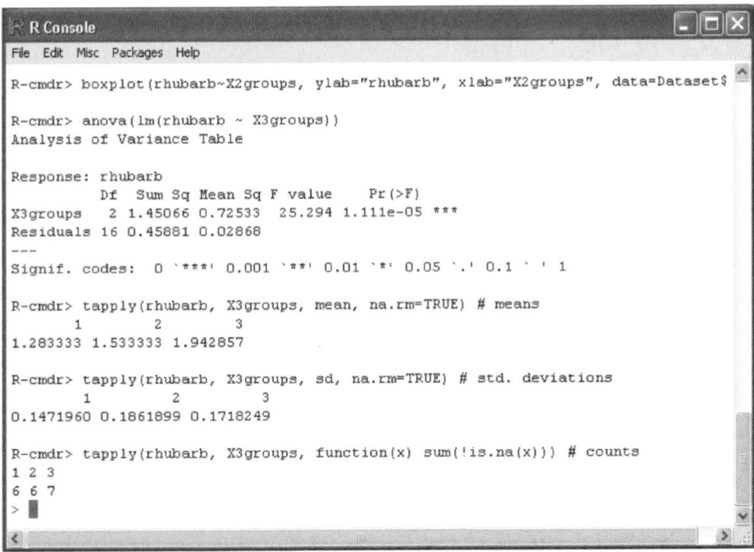

Fig. 7.14 ANOVA output.

Comparing two groups – chi-squared tests

Let's make another data-set. Once again, from the R Commander menu choose **Data** → **New Data Set**. Call this set *ChisqData*. This time we're seeing whether the gender of a participant makes it more or less likely that they are wearing grey flannel underwear. Enter the data – 40 observations (no, I'm not sure how they were made) for variables flannel (0 = grey, 1 = other) and gender (0 = male, 1 = female). Of the 20 males 14 had grey flannels on, but of the 20 females only seven had grey flannels on. Once you've finished, close the data editor window as before.

Note that when you're naming the variables (click at the top of each column) don't forget to tell R they are character variables (i.e. categorical) – a flannel value of 0.5 is meaningless in this context.

Next, still in R Commander, click on **Statistics** → **Contingency Tables** → **2-Way Tables**, choose the two variables flannel and gender, ensure the **Chi Square** test box is ticked, and click **OK**. Once again, the output is in the R Console and the syntax to ask the R Console to do the test directly is displayed in the R Console, if you scroll up and down. In the R Console you can also see a little table of the counts, which you can use to check you entered the data correctly.

As you can see, there is a significant gender difference: $P = 0.02667$, meaning there is a less than 3% probability that you obtained these results by pure chance. Women shun grey flannels, compared with men. Perhaps people will believe you now…

Conclusion

This is not a manual on study design, statistics or software, but it perhaps is somewhere to start from. Following these instructions you can at least have a go at performing a power calculation, entering data into a data-set, saving the analysis, summarising the data, generating a graph or two and performing some basic significance tests required for a simple research project. Moreover, this is all with a statistics package that is flexible, well supported, easy to use and, in the case of R, free!

CHAPTER 8

Reference management software

James Woolley

'The secret to creativity is knowing how to hide your sources.'
Albert Einstein (1879–1955)

Do you have trouble keeping track of references? Is your desk cluttered with stacks of journal papers? Ever wondered whether it is possible to keep track of new evidence automatically, electronically and in an easily accessible, searchable format? Making a database of ever-changing lists like this is just the sort of application computers are supposed to be good at, but until recently the software has had too steep a learning curve for widespread use. However, this is no longer true, and by the end of this chapter you should have a good understanding of what reference management software can achieve and how to use it to your advantage, and will see how easily it could be integrated into your daily work. In the words of Florynce Kennedy (1916–2000), 'Don't agonize. Organize!'

Even as a busy clinician, it is likely that you will have been asked to talk on topics that require at least a brief literature search to ensure that you are up to date. Reference management software has been developed primarily to help you to organise and retrieve your literature for research, teaching and publications. It is at its best when asked to create bibliographies in a variety of publication styles – and can even do this in real time as you type in your word processor ('cite while you write'). However, you could also use it as a friendly database to help index electronic resources as diverse as consultant contact details, patient information sheets and an electronic book (eBook) library.

Imagine having immediate, fully searchable access to reprint collections of journal papers, and the ability to compile reading lists for courses with a few button presses, or even to generate a list of authors' addresses and email addresses quickly and easily. It may be that you can keep this sort of information in your head, or at least know where (roughly) it is in your office, but the moment it reaches a certain critical mass, or needs sharing with someone else, that informal system may be found wanting. Reference management software allows you to search and sort *huge* databases of references (thousands, in seconds, across multiple subject areas).

The software also aids collaborative working with colleagues. Perhaps you are working on a paper together, but keep your references separately, in different formats, which gives the potential for no end of confusion, misunderstanding and duplication of effort. Reference management software would allow you to use a common format to exchange references, or even keep just one easily updated primary reference source between you. On a more pragmatic level, it also offers a solution to the seemingly deliberate policy of different journals to require references in subtly different formats, forcing you into tedious manual reformatting when your first choice rejects you. Now, you can just select the title of your second (third, fourth or eventually fifth) choice, watch your references instantly reformatted before your eyes, print them out and resubmit your paper to the next journal.

What does reference management software do?

Traditionally, researchers and writers spent hours filling in index cards, photocopying, filing and typing bibliographies. Essentially, the task was one of finding and collecting references, indexing and storing them before reproducing them in a different format. Reference management software can help integrate these processes and is now coming of age, with improved integration of the software with word processors and online databases. Using just a reference management software package, you can now:

- search a remote bibliographic database on the internet (such as Medline, PsychInfo or PubMed)
- import to your computer references of interest, creating your own personal reference library
- search within your database for any keywords or authors
- create independent bibliographies
- cite any of your references in a word-processed document, and create an instant bibliography formatted specifically for any of thousands of publications.

More advanced users can also make use of Microsoft Word templates for many journals, and even electronically store complete copies of journal articles for reading later. These can be retrieved with a simple search on a PC, thus helping to dispense with the piles of journal papers spilling over desks and clogging up drawers.

What is a reference?

As a starting point, it is worth noting that any reference can have many pieces of information ('fields'), in addition to the familiar author, paper and journal titles, date, issue and volume numbers, page numbers and abstract. These could include alternative titles or journals, labels, keywords, accession numbers, chapter titles, web links and even book covers. You may not use any of these routinely, but it can be very helpful to have them recorded for later reference.

Choosing reference management software

There are three widely known commercial packages: Reference Manager, EndNote and ProCite. In recent years they have all been acquired by the same company (ISI ResearchSoft: *http://www.isiresearchsoft.com*). These three products are gradually converging in terms of features, functionality and price, so the choice is largely a matter of personal preference. Versions of EndNote and ProCite are available for both Windows PCs and Apple Macs, whereas Reference Manager is only suitable for Windows. However, they are not cheap options: a typical individual user licence can cost from around £70 with an academic discount up to £300 for personal use. Many other developers produce software which may well suit your needs better (and more cheaply). There are too many of these packages to review here, but a visit to their websites should allow you to get a good feel for what is available (see Table 8.1 for some examples). If all this seems too overwhelming, there are websites that compare the features of most packages head-to-head. A good example is *http://www.burioni.it/forum/ors-bfs/index.html*, which is updated up to four times a year to keep pace with software developments.

Table 8.1 Examples of reference management software

Package	Website
Citation 8	http://www.citationonline.net
Library Master	http://www.balboa-software.com
Biblioscape	http://www.biblioscape.com/index.html
ResourceMate	http://www.resourcemate.com
Papyrus (free to download and use)	http://www.researchsoftwaredesign.com
GetARef	http://www.getaref.com
Bookends (for Mac only)	http://www.sonnysoftware.com
SquareNotes (free to download and use)	http://sqn.com/sqn5.html
Sixpack (for Linux)	http://www.santafe.edu/~dirk/sixpack/

There are also shareware packages (for which the user pays a small fee, usually £20–£30) and freeware packages (unsurprisingly, available at no cost). These have also evolved greatly, to the point where, unless your needs are especially complex, they are likely to be more than adequate for most users. As usual, the greatest choice is for users of Microsoft Windows, but there are good, well-featured products also for Apple and UNIX systems. Have a look at SquareNotes for an example of a free program for Windows, and for Linux users there is a set of Perl scripts called Sixpack, which can even be installed onto Windows if you are an advanced user (Table 8.1).

OpenOffice

This is a fully featured suite of programs (word processor, spreadsheet, presentation maker, etc.) that rivals Microsoft Office and is completely free (see Chapter 1). It already offers some bibliographic database functions (look in the **Tools** menu) and the existing commercial packages such as EndNote are partially able to integrate with it. The team behind OpenOffice is also planning to develop their own reference management software, which is likely to be as fully functional as the current commercial packages, but will be free (*http://bibliographic.openoffice.org/developer.html*).

Web-based reference managers

These are not installed as software on your computer, but rather accessed on the internet using your usual web browser (such as Internet Explorer or Firefox – see Chapter 10). This means your references are held in a personal account, rather like Hotmail or *doctors.net* emails, which you can access from any computer (Windows, Mac or UNIX) with internet access. An example is Refworks (*http://www.refworks.com/*), for which there is an annual subscription, or WriteNote from the makers of EndNote, Reference Manager and ProCite (*http://www.writenote.com*). Those of you with the good fortune to work in NHS Scotland or at certain academic institutions throughout the UK can access Refworks free via the NHS e-library (*http://www.elib.scot.nhs.uk*) – just speak to your local librarian for details.

Handheld computers

Reference management software is increasingly appearing for these popular machines. Users of palm and pocket PCs are catered for by many possibilities, from an Endnote file viewer to the free BiblioExpress (*http://www.biblioscape.com/biblioexpress.htm*) program. Qcite (*http://www.users.globalnet.co.uk/~dhenshaw/Qcite.htm*) can be used by Psion owners to organise references in a very sophisticated way for such a small gadget. New software is being developed all the time, so it is worth regularly checking search engines such as *http://www.google.com* or *http://www.tucows.com* for new programs.

Using reference management software

Despite the wide choice, most packages function in a similar way. We will now walk through some of the tasks you are most likely to want to try, for the sake of this exercise illustrated by the commands and screens used in EndNote.

Creating an EndNote Library

Creating an EndNote library is just like creating any other file or document (see Chapter 1). On the menu, click **File** → **New**. Enter a name for your new library and choose where to save it before clicking **File** → **Save**. EndNote library file names are automatically given the extension *.enl* (for EndNote library). The file name you enter appears in the top-left corner of the window. At the bottom-left corner of the window it will say 'Showing 0 out of 0 references', to show that your new EndNote library is empty.

Opening a library

On first starting the program, a box appears that allows you to open a reference 'library' (i.e. a computer file that holds references – you could have just one enormous reference list with everything, or a different library of references for each project). Choose **Open An Existing Library** and browse to the desired library. You can also open a library by clicking **File** → **Open** in the menu at the top of the screen. For example, I have a library file called *neuroimaging in schizophrenia*. Figure 8.1 shows what this looks like when opened.

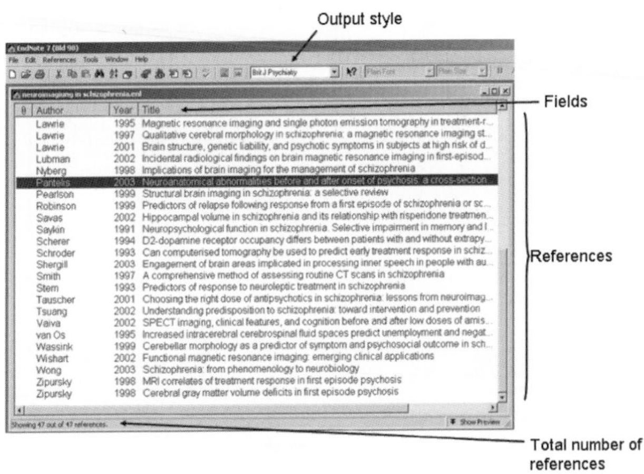

Fig. 8.1 An EndNote library file.

Sorting, finding and previewing references

You change the order in which references are displayed by clicking on the column (field) headings. If you click on the same heading twice, the references will be sorted in reverse order. To find a reference, you can:

- scroll through the list by using the arrow keys on your keyboard
- drag the vertical scroll bar at the right of your reference list up or down
- type the first few letters of the field by which the library is sorted (for example, if you clicked the title heading to sort the library by title, type the first few letters of a title to find that reference).

To see a preview of a reference in the output style you have currently selected, select an individual reference by clicking on it, then click **Show Preview** at the bottom right of your reference list (Fig. 8.2). To hide the preview, click **Hide Preview**.

Viewing a reference

To view a complete reference, double click on its line in the library, or click once and press [Enter]. The Reference window appears. This window allows you to view, enter or edit information for any field for a reference. You can also use this window to input new references into your library by hand (but before you do so, wait until you've read on to see how to do it automatically). You can also customise fields so that they hold other files

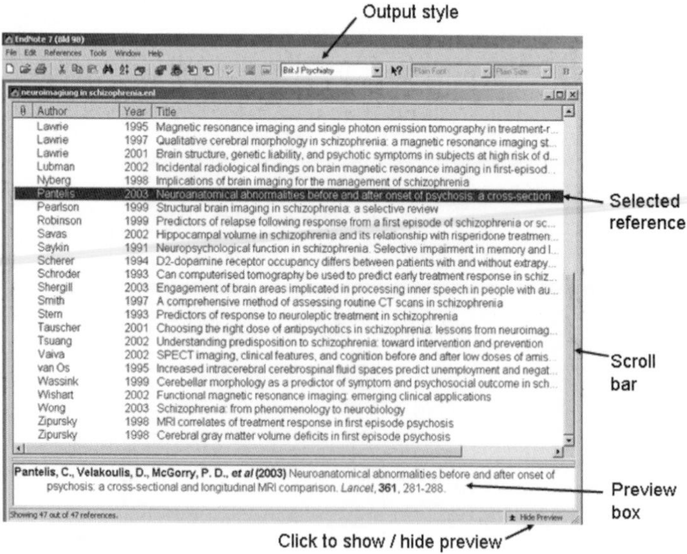

Fig. 8.2 Preview of references.

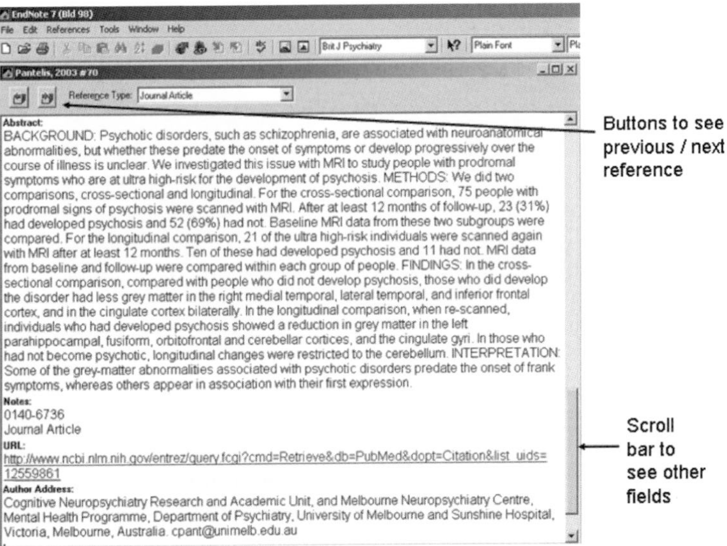

Fig. 8.3 Viewing references.

relating to the reference, such as a picture of cover of the book to which the reference refers, or an Acrobat (*.pdf*) file of a full journal article, thereby building your own virtual library.

Once you have created a database you can sort it using various fields, such as year of publication or author, with a single click. You may not want to see every single field about your references (such as ISBN or publisher), in which case it is simple to choose which fields are displayed (Fig. 8.3).

'Term lists' allow you to enter and reference articles consistently. They can consist of author names and keywords that will allow you to retrieve articles more efficiently. You can set these lists up yourself, or some packages spot patterns in previously entered references and suggest terms to you. They may even have predefined term lists for specific subjects, which could give you a head start.

You can search through your references for a specific word in just one field, or use wildcard characters to broaden your search over every field.

Adding references to a library

There are three ways to add references to an EndNote library:

- manually
- using EndNote's direct-connection feature to search remote databases
- importing references from other programs or downloading them from remote databases.

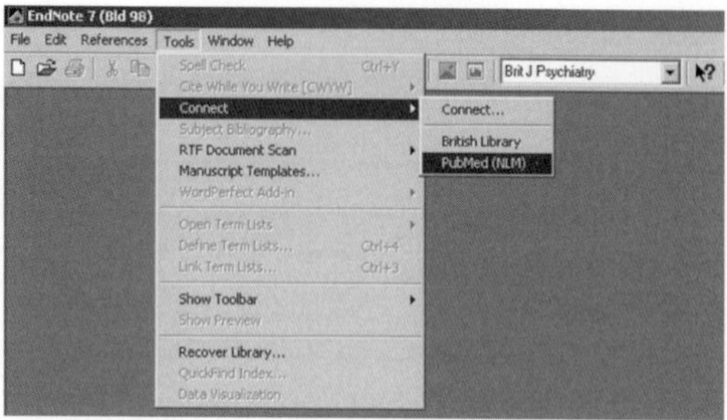

Fig. 8.4 Connecting to Medline.

Manually

We have already mentioned the manual option, and if you really want to do this, click **References → New Reference** to be presented with a long list of fields to fill in by hand. You may have to do this for non-published references, such as websites or lectures, so to help with this there is a drop-down box for selecting the reference type. This then ensures only the relevant fields are displayed for you to fill in. However, building your library electronically is much more efficient and accurate.

Direct connection to remote databases

This feature allows you to search remote databases over the internet from within EndNote. The example database we will use (see Fig. 8.4) is PubMed (Medline, hosted by the National Library of Medicine in the USA) at *http://www.nlm.nih.gov/*, but you can use many others.

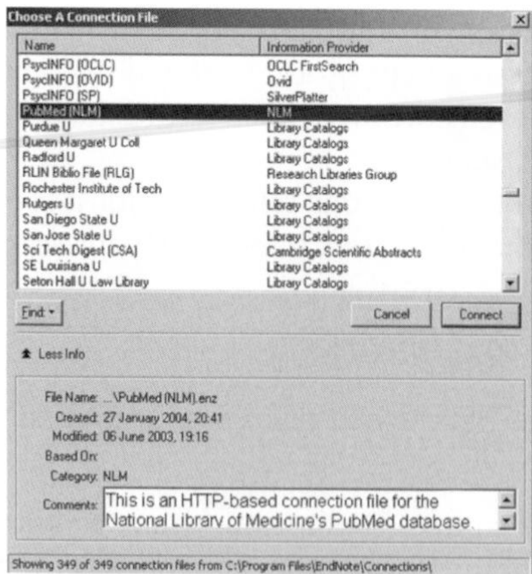

Fig. 8.5 Connection dialogue box.

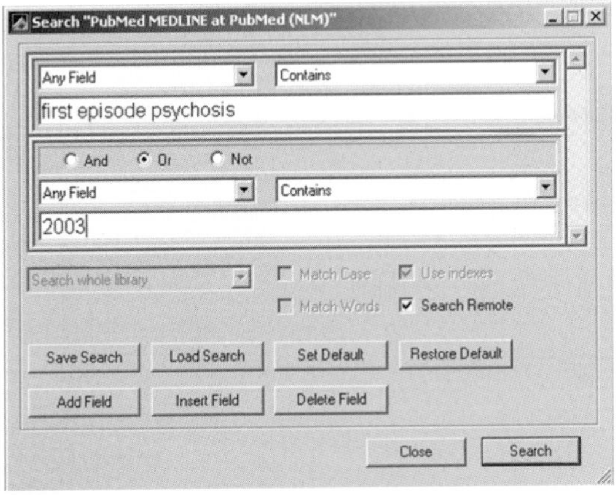

Fig. 8.6 Search fields.

Click **Tools** → **Connect** and a sub-menu appears (Fig. 8.5). Click the top item on the side menu **Connect...** for a full list of available databases. The other items in this menu are databases you have searched before, so you could just click on one to go straight back to it. A box appears to show a list of 'connection files' (databases you can connect to and search). To connect to a database, click on its name and click **Connect**. A box appears, with the name of the database at the top, that allows you to search within that database.

Enter your search text in one or more search fields, link them using standard Boolean (*and*, *or*, *not*) operators, and click **Search** to search the database. In the example shown in Fig. 8.6, **Title** was chosen using the drop-down menu, the **And** button was clicked and a publication year (2003) was entered. The search retrieved references containing the keyword phrase 'first episode psychosis' that were published in 2003. A **Confirm Remote Search** box appears (Fig. 8.7). Click **OK** to retrieve references and they will be downloaded from the internet, placed in a temporary file and displayed.

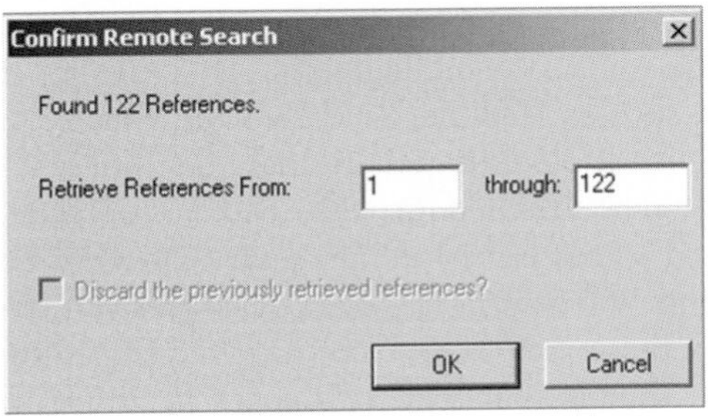

Fig. 8.7 Confirm remote.

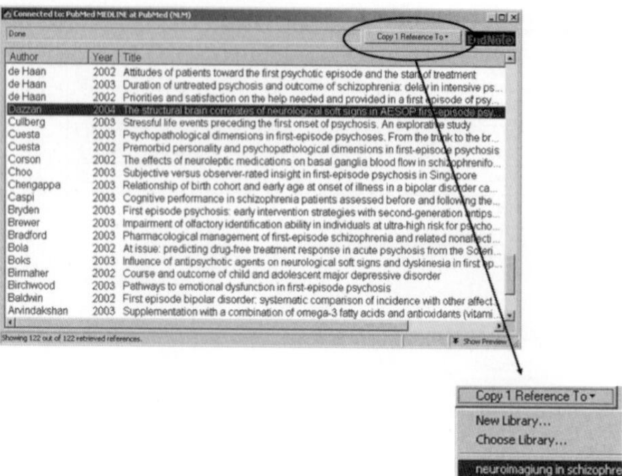

Fig. 8.8 Copy remote references.

Select the references you want to copy to your own EndNote library. (If you don't select any, then they will all be copied.) Click on the **Copy References To** drop-down menu, and choose the EndNote library to which you want to copy the references (Fig. 8.8).

And that's it! With these few steps, you have performed a journal search on every Medline-indexed paper publisher over a period of almost 40 years, refined it down to papers of specific interest and copied to your own reference library every identifying field you are ever likely to need. You have created an electronic, searchable abstract of each paper, all stored in a form that your word processor can use to output as a bibliography in the required style for any of thousands of journals.

Importing references

The above method of assembling references is the approach to take when you are starting from scratch, but don't worry if you have previously saved references from other databases (for example CD-ROM versions of Medline by SilverPlatter or Ovid). The third method is to 'import' citations you have saved from previous database searches into EndNote.

There are numerous bibliographic databases for many potential areas of interest, such as Medline, PsychInfo and Cinahl. Any of these can then be offered in various different formats for different users. For example, Medline could be searched through Ovid, SilverPlatter, ISI Web Of Science, PubMed and so on, either online or on CD-ROM. Local library licensing arrangements will determine which databases you can access.

The way these various services have developed over the past 20 years means that they format their references in different, often incompatible ways. Solving this is another strength of reference management software.

Most packages are able to import references from a huge range of databases for different formats, often using an 'import filter' specific to each database, which tells it how to insert the various fields into your personal database.

In EndNote, this function can be found in the main menu under **File → Import**. The precise method depends on the format in which your old references are saved, but a series of boxes guide you through the process of selecting the correct import filter in order to access your data. It even checks to make sure imported references don't duplicate your existing data.

Choosing an output style

Output styles allow you to change the format of your references with a single click. This is very useful if, for example, you submit an article to several different publishers, each of which has different formatting requirements for references. Output styles define the format of citations within the main text of a paper as well as within bibliographies, and EndNote comes preloaded with the required formats of thousands of journals. The easiest way to select an output style is to use the **Output Styles** drop-down menu on the right side of EndNote's main toolbar (Fig. 8.9).

By default, the **Output Styles** menu displays the **Annotated**, **Author-Date**, **Numbered** and **Show All** output styles. It also remembers styles you have used previously by adding them to the drop-down list. You can select output styles that are not in the list by clicking **Select another style** and scrolling down the list until you find the one you want; then click **Choose** and in future it will appear in your **Output Styles** drop-down menu. The new output style is reflected in the reference preview in the Endnote library window.

Instant bibliographies

Reference management software increasingly integrates with word processors, allowing you to select references for inclusion in a bibliography from within the word document itself ('cite while you write' – see Fig. 8.10). Having selected a citation within the main body of the text, it appears at the end of your document, correctly formatted for the selected journal.

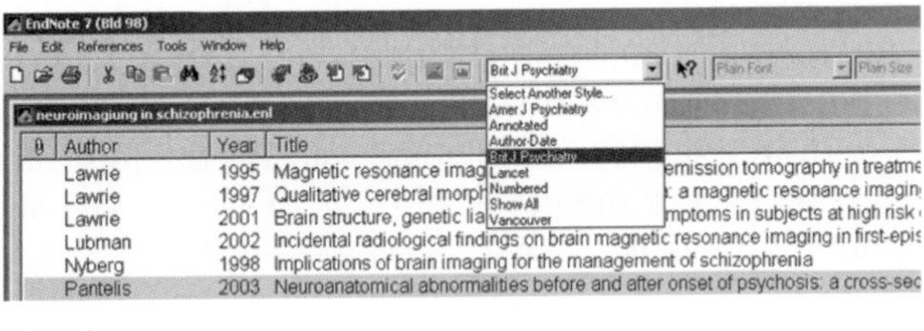

Fig. 8.9 Output styles.

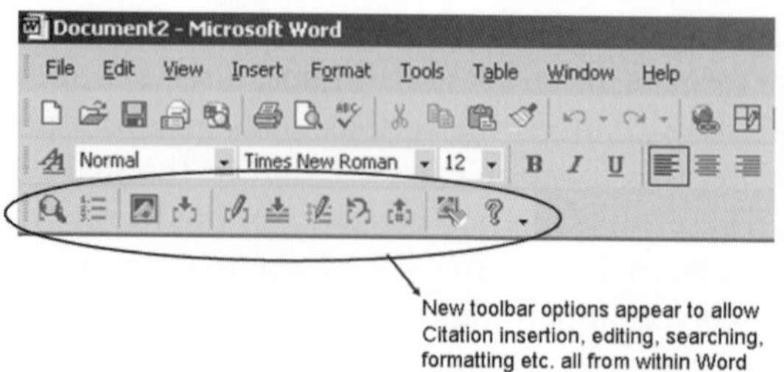

Fig. 8.10 'Cite as you write'.

Individual citations can be added, removed or reordered within the text at any time, and the bibliography automatically updates and (if appropriate) renumbers itself. If your intended publisher shows less interest than you had initially hoped, then simply changing the journal selection automatically reformats the citations and references throughout your entire document to the style required by the new journal, with a single click.

This integration with word processors is progressing, with some packages now including word processor template documents specific to various journals as well. So, at the outset, having selected a predefined template, the word processor prompts you for each element of the manuscript in correct sequence and formulates the bibliography and the figure list in a journal-specific format.

'Cite while you write' also allows you to insert images or figures contained within an EndNote library into a Microsoft Word document from within Word. They appear in parentheses in the main text, for example as '(Figure 1)', with the image itself appearing below the citation or at the end of the document (in a figures list). Again, this depends on the format style you currently have selected.

Conclusion

You should now have a better feel for what reference management software is, what it can do and, most importantly, how it may be useful to you. The steps we have covered should allow you to find your way round most of the available packages but, as with any software, there really is no substitute for getting stuck in and having a go – remember that at the end of the learning curve is the nirvana of a journal-free desk and drawers. Most companies provide free trial versions of their software, so why not go along to some of their websites and download some you like the look of? Even if you use only a fraction of the power of these programs, you should at least be able to avoid hearing yourself saying 'Now, I had a paper about that somewhere…'

CHAPTER 9

Mobile computing

Fionnbar Lenihan and Matt Evans

Mobile computing devices come in a range of shapes and sizes guaranteed to overload any classificatory scheme. The categorisation of mobile devices we use in this chapter is therefore somewhat arbitrary. Like the classification of personality disorder, it makes no claim to 'carve nature at the joints' but may be of some use to busy people at the front line.

We have chosen to look at mobile computing as a spectrum: at one end there is the 'Everest expedition' traveller, laden down with all the equipment that *might* be needed; at the other lies the 'hunter-gatherer', who travels the world with only a few passwords on a piece of paper. In between, we have intermediate solutions like personal digital assistants (PDAs) and smartphones. There is no one best spot on this spectrum, just trade-offs and compromises. In this chapter, we aim to help you find ones that you can live with.

Sub-notebooks and tablets

The first point on our spectrum of mobility is conceptually the easiest. A sub-notebook is merely a laptop that has, by dint of clever engineering, been miniaturised. It runs the same operating system (OS) and applications as a 'real' computer – because it is a 'real' computer. While small, the keyboards on these machines are usually good enough for touch typing and the screens are relatively easy to read. You can use your existing skills and there are no awkward issues about keeping the data on the mobile device consistent with your main computer ('synchronisation'), since the sub-notebook will probably be your main computer.

What, then, are the inevitable trade-offs with sub-notebooks?

A miniature laptop will generally cost more than a similarly specified 'regular' laptop, thereby making it an attractive target for thieves and more expensive to insure.

Compared with a desktop, or even a normal laptop, a sub-notebook will be slower, have less memory, less hard disk storage and less impressive

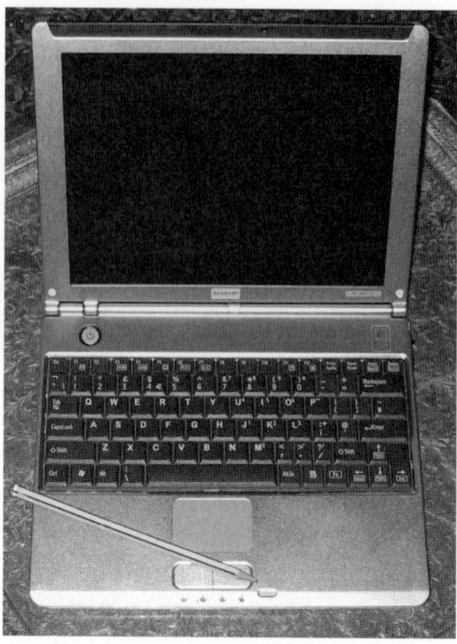

Fig. 9.1 A sub-notebook computer.

graphics cards. While the keyboard and screen will be usable, they may still be tiring and frustrating over long periods.

In the Windows world, the Sharp PC-MM1110 (Fig. 9.1) and the Sony Vaio are both highly desirable sub-notebooks. Apple's 12-inch PowerBook also fits into this category.

One recent variant on the sub-notebook theme is the so-called 'tablet' computer, which is in essence a sub-notebook that has a touch sensitive screen (see Chapter 2).

PDAs

Broadly speaking, PDAs can be grouped into palm and pocket PC devices (the two mainstream 'varieties') and a variety of 'other' devices. The palm devices run the Palm operating system (from Palm One), whereas the pocket PC devices run a superficially Windows-like operating system from Microsoft (by the time you read this it will probably be called Windows Mobile 2005). Other devices run operating systems such as Linux and Symbian. There are differences between these operating systems but for the palm and pocket PC devices at least, the functionality is most definitely converging. Before looking for the most appropriate device to meet your needs, it is important to understand some basic principles of the hardware, the mobile networking available on PDAs, and the software run on them.

PDA hardware options

Screen

In general, big screens are better than small ones and high resolution is better than low (resolution is the number of dots comprising the display). Colour depth is another factor: in general, the more colours the better. Bear in mind, though, that increases in these numbers can reduce both portability and battery life.

Input methods

Most PDAs have a touch-sensitive screen – that is, you can interact with the device by pressing on the screen, usually with a small plastic pen called a stylus. Using special key strokes, you can input text character by character. Some devices have a 'soft' or 'virtual' keyboard that appears on the screen, while others have a real (but very small) keyboard. Both are a bit fiddly and if you need to input a lot of information you should invest in a folding keyboard. These devices are themselves the size of a PDA when folded. Once unfolded, they have keys similar to those on a laptop computer. Wireless versions include the PocketTop keyboard (*http://www.pocketop.net*).

Battery life

Battery life can vary greatly. Setting the screen at full brightness or using wireless communications will rapidly drain any battery, so it is a good idea to check the manufacturer's quoted figure (usually a little optimistic) for battery life to ensure it will meet your needs. You should usually be able to use your PDA for a day or two before it needs to be recharged. Bear in mind that if you let your battery run down you may well lose *all* of the data on your machine. PDAs are usually recharged by placing them in the synchronisation cradle.

There are various devices to help keep your PDA charged, such as external battery packs, charging cables for computer USB ports or car lighter sockets and, most simply, a spare battery. Not every PDA, however, has batteries than can be swapped in this way.

The key is to make sure you back up your device regularly (daily if possible). Always back up before going away on holiday, as many PDAs will be completely drained of power after a week even without being used.

Storage slots

Most devices allow a memory card (Fig. 9.2) to be inserted to expand the storage available to the PDA so that more programs can be installed or more files stored. Common slot standards are the compact flash (CF) slot and the smaller secure digital/multimedia card slot (SD/MMC). Some PDAs have one of each type, which adds great versatility. In addition to memory cards, other accessories like modems, wireless cards and USB adapters have

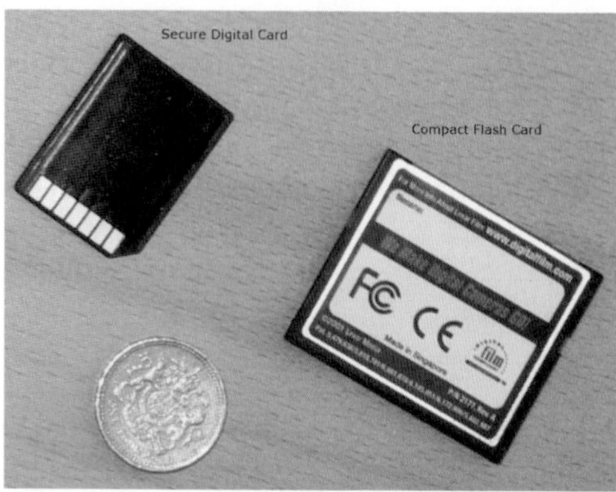

Fig. 9.2 Memory cards.

been designed to use these slots. You should think what you are likely to be using the PDA for in the future, as this will determine what type of slot and how many of them you will require.

Mobile networking for PDAs

This area can be quite confusing as there are so many competing standards. The following (simplified) definitions are given to help you try to make sense of the available options.

Infra-red

This rather old technology is still present on many PDAs and mobile phones. It works over short distances (i.e. centimetres rather than metres) and requires both infra-red ports (see Chapter 1) to have a clear line of sight.

Bluetooth

This is superior to infra-red because it operates over several metres and does not require a line of sight. For instance, a mobile phone in a briefcase could receive a signal from a PDA on a desktop. Bluetooth can be used for many purposes, such as connecting a phone to a PDA or a headset to a phone, or to send documents wirelessly to a printer.

WiFi ('wireless LAN')

This is similar technology to Bluetooth but has a greater range. It is used primarily to replace the cables used in local area networks (LANs) such as you might find in a business or hospital. It is also used to make connections to the internet, either over wireless LANs in people's homes or at 'hotspots', such as in coffee shops and airports, where you can pay to be allowed access to a fast internet connection. Security of information is important since your files or internet activity are being beamed around the place. The encryption protocol WEP and the safer WPA should reduce the chance of your information ending up in the wrong hands and you are advised to ensure that this security is enabled.

Mobile phone communications

Some PDAs have built-in mobile phones, while others make use of infrared, Bluetooth or a cable to connect to the mobile phone. Once your device can connect to a mobile phone it can then access the internet. The method it uses will depend on the type of hardware you have as well as the services available from the phone company (Fig. 9.3). The simplest is a dial-up connection via the phone. The PDA needs to have a modem to send and receive the data via the phone and uses a normal (GSM) low-speed connection running at about 9600 bits per second (9.6 kbps). While this may be adequate for a few emails, large file transfers will take a long time. Since this type of connection is charged by the minute, you might also find it expensive.

Another type of data connection is GPRS (General Packet Radio Service). This is an always-on connection – once the phone is connected, the link

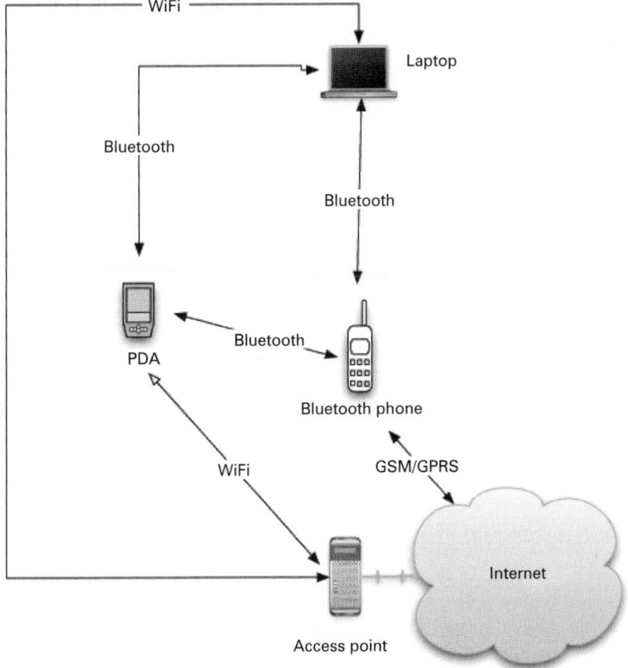

Fig. 9.3 Mobile wireless.

remains open. The speed is approximately 56 kbps and the charge is usually by the kilobyte or as part of a data bundle (a certain amount of data is permitted 'free' every month). This method is far more suitable for email, web browsing and some file transfers but be aware that it can be easy to run up a large phone bill if your data use is high.

Currently the fastest means of data connection over a mobile phone network is 3G. This operates at about 384 kbps, which is about as fast as a slow broadband connection. Costs are still very high, however. Most mobile phone networks now offer a 3G mobile modem that fits into the card slot of a laptop.

Software options for PDAs

Core applications

All modern PDAs come with a core set of built-in programs, which you are likely to use most. These include a calendar (Fig. 9.4), to-do list (Fig. 9.5), address book and a jotter. You will sometimes hear these referred to as PIM (personal information management) applications. (We will try to spare you further TLAs – three-letter acronyms!)

The PIM applications on different devices are broadly similar, so choice is largely a matter of personal taste. However, if you plan to synchronise (see below) your PDA with a main computer (and you should), then you need to make sure that the PDA and the computer can talk to one another. In general, Microsoft PDAs talk only to Microsoft operating systems and Microsoft applications (like Outlook), so if, for example, you use a Mac or a PIM program like Lotus Organiser on a Windows machine you might have difficulties.

Be aware also that keeping patient information on your personal PDA may give rise to issues of confidentiality and data protection. David Harris has more to say on this in Chapter 12.

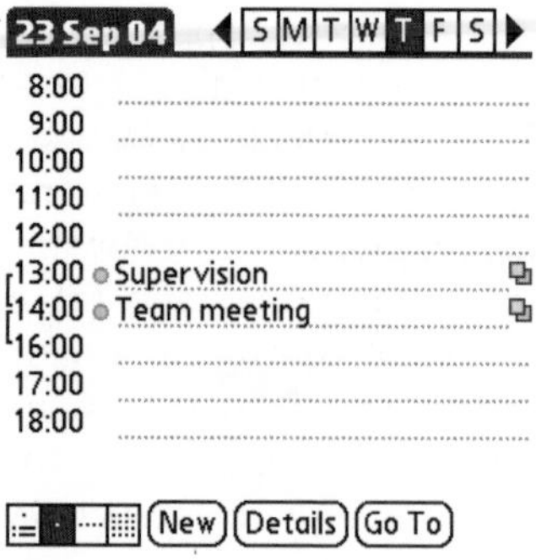

Fig. 9.4 The palm calendar.

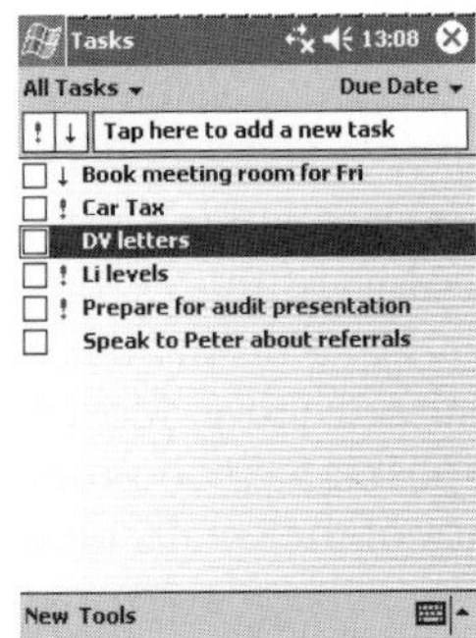

Fig. 9.5 The pocket PC to-do list.

All the core applications can be 'synchronised' with your desktop PC. This means that when you connect your PDA with your main PC (either by putting it in the supplied cradle or over a wireless connection) it will update any changes made in both directions. Thus, the PDA is backed up and the dates, to-do items and so on can be accessed on the full-size computer. Generally, you can synchronise with more than one PC and it is possible to mark appointments as being private or business related so that the synchronisation program knows whether or not to synchronise each item to a given machine.

Office applications

Word processing, spreadsheets and databases together comprise this category. Surprisingly, their importance on the desktop is not matched in the PDA field. Chiefly this is because of the inherent limitations of screen size and input method. There are contrary views but, in our experience, large amounts of text input are best done on a desktop or laptop, with the PDA used for minor edits on the move.

The pocket versions of both Word and Excel bundled with a pocket PC are feeble, so if you do want to use your PDA for creating large documents or spreadsheets on the move you should probably upgrade to TextMaker and PlanMaker respectively (for the pocket PC). These can be bought and downloaded from *http://www.softmaker.de/tmp_en.htm*. Most palm PCs come with Documents To Go, and the excellent WordSmith from Blue Nomad Software (*http://www.bluenomad.com*) is available as a downloadable trial version.

A database program, in contrast, really makes sense on a PDA. In addition to the obvious use of storing information, a portable database application is very useful for data capture, say for a survey or audit. The screens or forms into which you enter data can be customised so that options can be selected from menus rather than laboriously entered by hand. Furthermore, a good database package can give you much of the power of programming without the need to learn any code (see Chapter 6).

HanDBase (no, it's not a typo) from DDH software (*http://www.ddhsoftware.com*) is, in our view, an excellent database application for both palm and pocket PCs. Databases can easily be exchanged between the two types of PDA and there is a large library of ready-made databases, many medical, available at the DDH website.

Email is available on most PDAs now and is a major reason for using the networking technology discussed above. Most email applications on PDAs will synchronise with your desktop email program (e.g. Outlook), so that the PDA will contain a mirror of the emails on your desktop machine. This is useful for catching up on emails outside the office. You can reply to the emails and then choose to send them immediately or the next time the PDA synchronises.

Internet applications

Special browser programs enable you to have full access to the web from a PDA, although the small size of the screen makes it somewhat tricky to view certain sites. The best sites to look at are the ones specifically designed for PDAs (e.g. with few graphics). Even if the information you want isn't available in a PDA-friendly website, most PDA browsers will do their best to split the page up into columns so that you only have to scroll up and down to read them rather than side to side as well. A number of applications will use your main PC to download web content that you specify and package it up so that it can be viewed offline on your PDA. Many will do this automatically when you synchronise, so you can obtain pages from, say, the *BMJ*, the *British Journal of Psychiatry* or BBC News and read them at your leisure. Try the following services or software:

- *http://www.avantgo.com*
- *http://www.sitescooper.org*
- *http://www.plkr.org*

Miscellaneous applications

It is surprisingly easy to get engrossed in a book stored on a PDA, although our personal preferences will always be for paper. Many types of document can be read on a PDA so long as you have the appropriate software, which in many cases is free (Adobe Acrobat Reader, MS.lit files, Palm Reader, doc files, mobipocket and others). Try *http://www.memoware.com* for a wide selection of e-books in different formats.

It is now possible to hold a street map of the entire UK (including house numbers and all UK postcodes) on a PDA (Fig. 9.6). This can be incredibly useful in a meeting of the community mental health team when allocating home visits or resolving catchment area disputes. Furthermore, the same software can be used alongside a global positioning system (GPS costs approximately £100 to £200) so that it will voice navigate you in the car (or on foot) as well as displaying a moving three-dimensional map while

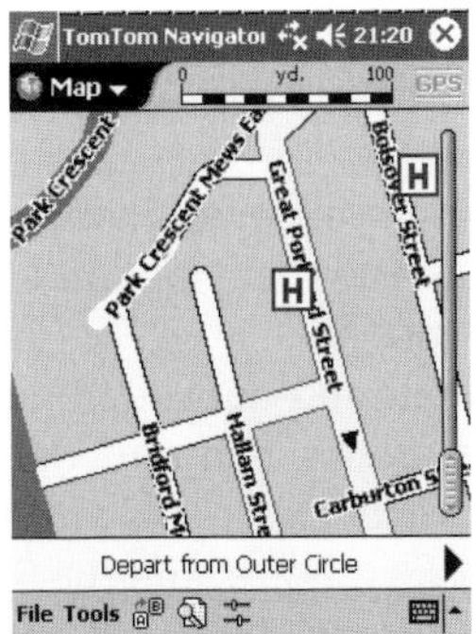

Fig. 9.6 Navigation software.

you are on your way. Try *http://www.tomtom.com* for software available on both palm and pocket PCs and *http://www.pocketgpsworld.com* for general information on available options.

Conclusion

We have only touched the surface regarding potential uses of PDAs. References such as ICD–10, DSM–IV, guidelines from the National Institute for Health and Clinical Excellence (NICE) and the *British National Formulary* (BNF) can be bought and a free drug database for palm PCs is available from *http://www.epocrates.com*. You can even download the contents of the *British Journal of Psychiatry* each month from *http://bjp.rcpsych.org*. Much software is available free or at a reasonable price. Sites like *http://www.handango.com* and *http://www.pocketgear.com* are good places to start looking and *http://www.brighthand.com* is a good source for news on PDA developments.

Smartphones

Most people do not realise that highly portable, networked computers are already ubiquitous in most developed countries. We are, of course, referring to mobile phones, which have, over the years, incorporated increasingly computer-like features.

The main advantage of an all-in-one device is, obviously, that you get to carry one fewer gadgets around with you. Since mobile phones are, by definition, connected to a network, access to email and the internet is potentially much easier and less fiddly using a combined device than with a phone and separate PDA. With clever design, the phone and PDA features of the one device can be made to work together in useful ways. Examples of this include having access to your entire address book when making phone calls and the ability to send notes, contacts or calendar appointments as emails or text (SMS) messages to anyone in your address book with a few key presses.

The main downside to smartphones is the fact that they are phones and as such subject to a range of restrictions, notably on-board aeroplanes, trains and in hospitals.

All the clever added features of smartphones also come at a price in terms of battery life and you may find that you don't get the same mileage as you did with your old 'dumb' phone.

It is fair to say that input and output are an even more acute problem for smartphones than for PDAs. Some models of smartphone have little keyboards, while some have touch screens on which you write. Others, such as the Windows Mobile smartphones and the Symbian Series 60 range (see below), require you to use predictive text from the number pad. While this may work for a short text message, it will soon become very tedious if you plan on producing longer documents or emails on the machine itself.

This can be worked around to some extent by doing intensive data entry on your main PC and relying on the synchronisation process (see under PDAs, above) to get the information across to your smartphone. To do this you will need to link the phone and the computer using an infra-red, Bluetooth or cable connection. Therefore make sure that your chosen model will work with your computer, operating system and diary/address book software. Windows and MS Outlook are usually supported and many phones will work with Apple machines also (see *http://www.apple.com/macosx/features/isync/devices.html* for a full listing in this regard).

Models

Below is a brief survey of the field of smartphones at the time of writing. Prices are not given, because they depend on the network package chosen.

Symbian

There are currently three main families of Symbian phones, the Series 60 range, Series 90 and the UIQ range. Series 60 handsets are more like traditional mobile phones and are designed to be operated with one hand, while the UIQ models are more like PDAs. The Series 90 phones have wide screens and are optimised for games and multimedia. All support infra-red and Bluetooth connectivity. The best way to get a feel for which type might suit you is to visit some phone shops and play with the demonstration models. See the Symbian home page at *http://my-symbian.com* for up-to-date news and *http://www.allaboutsymbian.com* for software.

Palm/Handspring

Palm and its former rival Handspring (recently acquired by Palm) are traditional PDA manufacturers, so it is not surprising that their products are more like PDAs than those from Symbian. The Treo range of smartphones resembles a traditional PDA with an antenna sticking out of the top. Unlike other Palm models, they have a small QWERTY keyboard, although

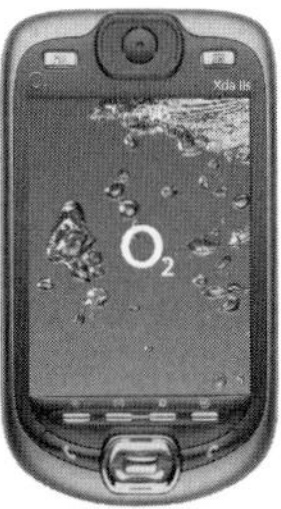

Fig. 9.7 The O2 XDA.

a touch-sensitive screen and stylus are still present. Because they share their hardware and operating system with other Palm PDAs, the Treo benefits from the enormous range of software available for that platform. You can find out more at *http://euro.palmone.com/uk/*.

Microsoft

Like Symbian, Microsoft takes two main approaches to creating a smartphone – bolt a phone on to a PDA or smarten up a conventional phone. The former approach (Pocket PC phone edition) gives you the O2 XDA/XDA II (Fig. 9.7), which is a conventional pocket PC (see above) with added phone capability. The latter approach is the one taken by the Windows Mobile smartphone, such as the Orange SPV.

Both the pocket PC phones and the Windows Mobile smartphones are designed to work best with other Microsoft products. If you use non-MS solutions such as Mac OS, Lotus Notes or Eudora you may be well advised to look elsewhere.

You can find out more about these Microsoft options at *http://www.microsoft.com/windowsmobile/default.mspx*.

Portable storage solutions

An informal survey of any train or plane will show that many people who bring a laptop end up stowing it in the overhead. In effect, they are interested in the computer only as a data store, to be used at the eventual destination. Why not take just the data and spare their backs?

Floppy disks are too small and too fragile to be useful data stores but recordable CD-ROM (CR-R) is an interesting option being very cheap and spacious (about 700 megabytes). Certainly, this is an excellent way to carry large presentations, graphics or other data that you don't expect to alter on the road. If, however, you want to edit your files away from base, you run into problems. Rewritable CD drives (CD-RW) are far from universal and often disks that work in one drive fail in another.

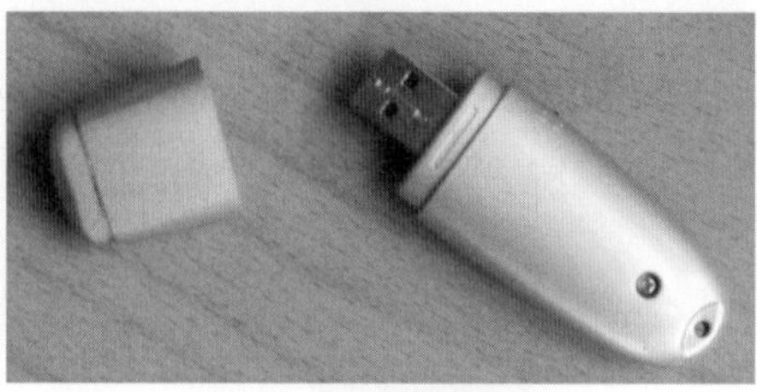

Fig. 9.8 A USB flash drive.

The past couple of years have seen a proliferation of small and relatively inexpensive storage devices based on so-called 'flash' memory. Variously called 'thumb drives', 'USB flash drives' or 'pen drives', these devices look like a highlighter pen (Fig. 9.8) and are currently available in a variety of sizes, from 8 megabytes up to 1 gigabyte.

Another option is to use one of the new breeds of music player. You may have seen (or lusted after) an Apple iPod. It is, however, only one of many portable music players (e.g. Archos, iRiver) that incorporate a hard disk drive (Fig. 9.9). In addition to storing a vast amount of music, this means that the player can also function as a portable external disk drive, with capacities shortly reaching 100 gigabytes. Unlike a flash-based drive, which will realistically transport only a selection of your files, a device with a hard disk offers the possibility of carrying a copy of *all* your files in your pocket.

The key to the success of both these portable storage solutions is the USB port. This is a standard port which is present and supported on Windows, Macintosh and Linux machines and which allows you to plug in a variety of devices. It is worth getting a USB2 device rather than the older 1.1 standard, as the transfer speed is many times faster. The flash or hard disk device is either plugged straight into the USB port of your computer or else the connection is made with a supplied cable. Typically there will be a beeping sound and the new device will show up on the desktop (Mac OSX), in 'My

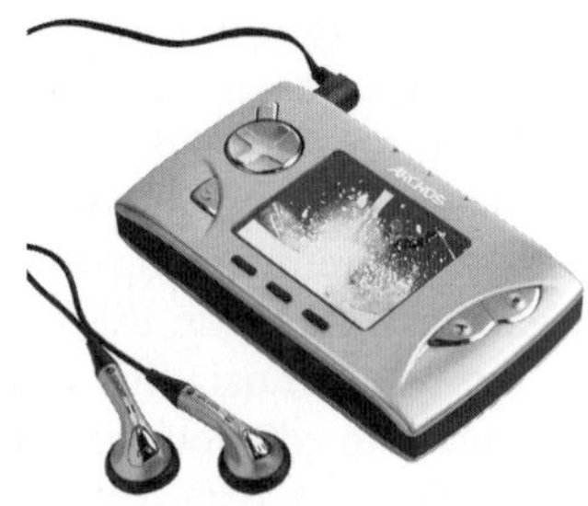

Fig. 9.9 Music player/portable hard drive.

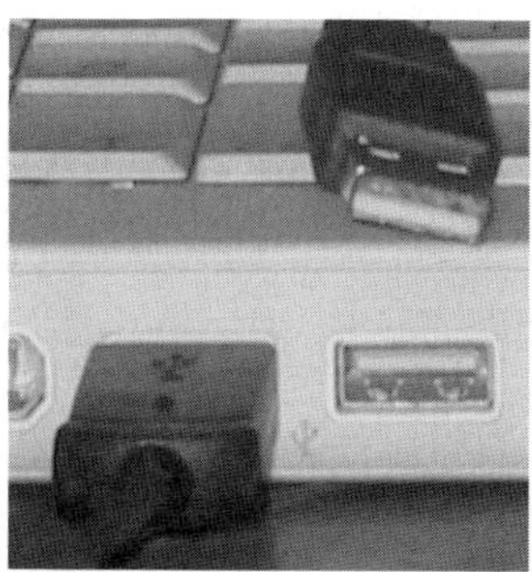

Fig. 9.10 USB port and connector.

Computer' (Windows) or God knows where (Linux). Both the USB cable and socket are adorned with the rather odd symbol shown (Fig. 9.10; see also Fig. 1.4, p. 3).

In this scenario, then, you would copy some or all of your files on to your portable device before hitting the road. At your destination you would borrow a computer (or use a cyber cafe), grab the files you needed from your storage device, work on them and copy the modified files back to your device. A hidden benefit of this approach is that there will always be two copies of your data hanging around as insurance against disaster. A hidden drawback is that, unless you are very careful, you will accumulate multiple versions of the same files as you copy them back and forth between systems. It is all too easy in this situation to overwrite a file with an earlier version of itself.

The briefcase utility bundled in most versions of Windows was designed to overcome this difficulty. To create a new briefcase, right click anywhere on the desktop. In the resulting pop-up menu chose **New → Briefcase**. A helpful wizard should now appear and guide you through the rest of the process. There is also a good tutorial at *http://www.support.microsoft.com/default.aspx?scid=kb;en-us;307885&sd=tech*.

The briefcase option works only between Windows machines. For a solution that works between Windows, Linux and (soon) Macs, you could try Unison (*http://www.cis.upenn.edu/~bcpierce/unison/*). Study the documentation carefully.

Apart from data, email is the main reason 'road warriors' carry their lumbar-popping burdens. Can portable storage displace the laptop here too? The answer is yes, at least if there is a machine at your destination with internet access. Popcorn (*http://www.ultrafunk.com/products/popcorn/*) is a shareware ($20) email program that will run entirely from any removable storage device. Simply plug in the storage device, wait until it is recognised, navigate to the device using Windows Explorer and double click on the Popcorn executable file (*popcorn.exe*). Mail will be saved to the device, not to the host computer, and once home the saved email can be imported into your main email program.

The Thunderbird email client that we will use as an example in Chapter 11 comes in a portable edition that can also be run from removable storage. Download this free and open-source application (see Preface) from *http://portablethunderbird.mozdev.org*.

'Living off the land'

In 1845, Sir John Franklin set off in HMS *Erebus* and HMS *Terror* to discover the fabled Northwest Passage. The two Royal Navy vessels were fabulously equipped by the standards of the time with china dinner services, pianos and several years' worth of tinned food. The whole expedition, however, died horribly, with its eventual fate ascertained by John Rae, a Scottish doctor who had learned the arts of snow-shoe travel and Arctic survival from the local Inuit peoples.

The point of this, slightly morbid, digression is to point out that packing for every conceivable eventuality does not necessarily represent wisdom. Most destinations in the developed world will have some information technology infrastructure that can be pressed into service.

For business travellers it may be possible to arrange a guest account at your destination in advance or, once there, someone may be kind enough to log you in (although this is to be frowned upon from a security point of view). Alternatively, your friends may let you use their computer, your hotel may have a business centre or there may be a convenient cyber cafe.

Email

Most internet users are probably familiar with Hotmail, the web-based email service from Microsoft that lets you check your mail from any internet-connected computer. The famous search company Google is currently launching a similar service, which features a very generous amount of storage and powerful search tools to 'Google' your archived mail.

You may, however, have a 'regular' (POP-compliant) email account, perhaps from your employer or your internet service provider. These, too, can be accessed over the internet using a web page such as *http://www.mail2web.com*. This service in effect logs into your mailbox for you and displays your mail as a web page. Using mail2web you can read, compose, reply, delete and forward mail and attachments. When you get home your mail is still on the POP server from where it can be downloaded into your mail program as usual.

Such services tend to have a relatively short business life. If you cannot access this site, go to a search engine such as Google and enter the search terms *web based pop access*. The results should contain some similar services.

Accessing files

Many companies provide internet-based file storage for a fee or free. The idea is that you store your files, or a subset of them, on the company's server. To access these files from a cyber cafe or other computer you simply go to the web page of the service and enter the username and password you were given when you joined. You will then be shown a list of all the files you have stored on the server, which you can retrieve, delete or add to via the web page. Some of these services have nifty software which, when run on your own PC, will make the web-based storage appear to be like a local hard drive (just very, very sloooow!). This of course won't be available to you when using someone else's PC.

Look at *http://www.freewebsiteproviders.com/virtual-disk-drives.htm* for a list of free storage providers or run a search in your favourite search engine for *web based file storage* or similar terms.

Online organisers

Companies such as Yahoo (*http://uk.yahoo.com*) and Schedule Online (*http://www.scheduleonline.com*) offer online calendars, address books and task managers. These resemble the corresponding applications on a PDA or smartphone and in some cases can be synchronised with such devices. It is possible to set up online organisers so that other people (such as your spouse or secretary) can view or modify your diary. If nothing else, these services act as a very useful backup to your PDA, saving your life from complete disintegration should it break or be stolen.

Words of caution

Mike Madden will be explaining the importance of security in Chapter 13, but it is worth noting at this point that the internet was never designed with security or confidentiality in mind and that patient-identifiable information should never be entrusted to online file storage services or posted on your online calendar. Even 'regular' email (outside your own local network) should not be used for clinical correspondence without approved encryption methods being used.

Computers typically hold temporary information stores or 'caches' in order to speed up internet activity. These will persist after you have finished your cappuccino and departed the cyber cafe, leaving your credit card number potentially retrievable. Similarly, 'deleted' files are not so much destroyed as de-indexed and can easily be restored.

Conclusion

Our intention in this chapter has been to give an overview of what mobile computing is all about. There is far more information to get across than can be fitted within a single chapter, so you are advised to follow up on the web links we have included or check out our website (*http://www.rcpsych.ac.uk/computers_and_internet_psychiatry*). When buying a PDA do have a look and even a 'play' with the different devices in shops or owned by colleagues. A second-hand or 'end of line' device might enable you to find out, at minimal expense, what you really require. There are also some very good current models available for as little as £100 which have all the core functions, so it is unlikely you will require the machines that cost £300 or more that the salespeople are so keen to sell you.

CHAPTER 10

Internet resources for psychiatrists

Gurpal Singh Gosall

The internet has probably been the biggest development in communications technology since the invention of television. The present, worldwide, computer network had its origins in the 1960s, when the US military began to link its different computer networks using common 'internet working' communications protocols (or rules).

Rapid expansion followed as academic departments and research institutions around the world discovered the benefits of shared computing resources and rapid electronic communication. By the early 1990s home users were able to access this 'information superhighway' and the popularity of the network became such that today it is hard to envisage life without it.

The internet is not run by any one organisation. Instead, it is a loosely organised series of independent computer networks, run by telecommunications companies, universities, research centres and private individuals, with no single network essential to the operation of the whole. Voluntary cooperation between these decentralised parties allows 'packets' of information to be exchanged across the network using the standard protocols referred to above. In this way, even computers with different processors and operating systems (see Chapters 1 and 2) can exchange information.

To most people, the internet means the 'World Wide Web', but this is a simplification. The underlying foundation of the internet is the Transmission Control Protocol/Internet Protocol, commonly abbreviated to TCP/IP. Web, email, Telnet, Usenet, File Transfer Protocol and other such network applications use their own protocols that lie 'on top of', or assume the existence of, TCP/IP.

The World Wide Web

The World Wide Web is a collection of specially formatted documents stored on internet servers, accessible via the internet and transmitted between computers using a protocol called HTTP (HyperText Transfer

Protocol). These documents are written in HTML (HyperText Mark-up Language), which supports hypertext links to other documents, graphics, audio and video files. Users can jump from one document to another by simply clicking on links displayed within each document. This allows for easy navigation of the web through the use of graphical user interfaces and links, and it is this feature that largely explains the explosive growth of the web since its development in 1989.

Web browsers

In order to access the World Wide Web, you must use a piece of software called a web browser, which can interpret HTML and display web pages correctly. The most common browser in use is Internet Explorer, from Microsoft (*http://www.microsoft.com/windows/ie*), but there are excellent alternatives such as the renowned Firefox (*http://www.mozilla.org/products/firefox/*) and Opera (*http://www.opera.com*).

For illustration purposes this chapter focuses on Internet Explorer, but the other options differ only in detail.

Using your browser

When you launch Internet Explorer or another web browser (see Chapter 1 for information on launching programs), the screen is divided into a number of areas (Fig. 10.1). Starting from the top, the *title* of the window is that of the website being browsed, in the example in Fig. 10.1, that of the Royal College of Psychiatrists. Below this is the *menu bar*, which gives you access to all the functions of the browser. Some of these functions are also shown below the menu bar, in the form of icons in the *toolbar*, allowing easier and faster access.

- The **Back** button returns you to the previous page you visited.
- The **Forward** button takes you to the next page you visited, if you are viewing recently visited pages.
- The **Stop** button stops the browser from downloading the current page.
- The **Refresh** button reloads the page you are viewing. You may wish to do this if the page was incompletely downloaded the first time or if the content changes, such as on a news page showing the latest football scores.
- The **Home** button takes you to your home page. If you haven't set a home page, you will see the default (standard) home page of your internet service provider or perhaps the Microsoft home page. You can change this by going to **Tools → Internet Options → General → Home Page**. For example, set it to *http://news.bbc.co.uk* to be greeted by the latest headlines from the BBC every time you start your browser or press

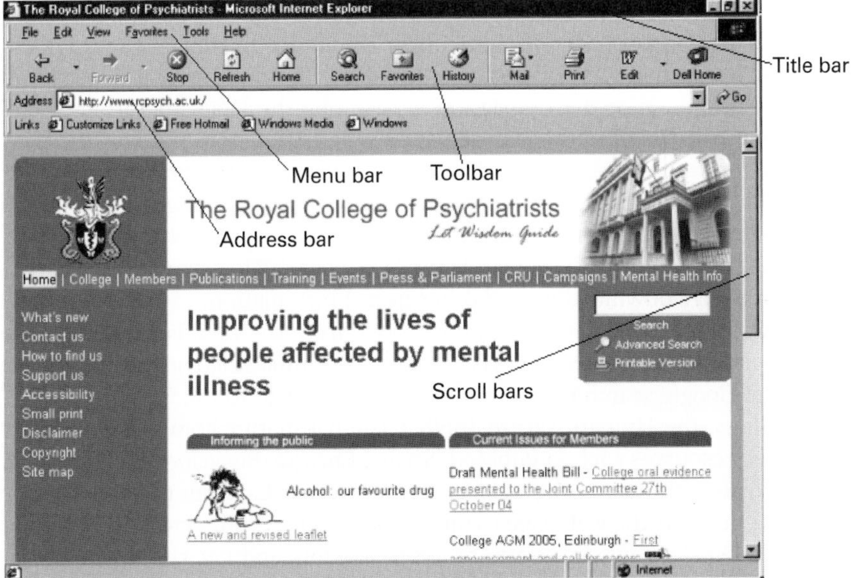

Fig. 10.1 The web browser.

the **Home** button. Many people set their home page to a search engine, such as *http://www.google.com* (see below on search engines).

- The next buttons along on the toolbar open up task panes in which additional information is shown. The **Search** button allows you to search the web while displaying a web page, the **Favorites** button shows you the websites that are in your list of favourites and lets you add to it, and the **History** button lists websites you have recently visited. You can sort the history list by date, by website name, by order of visiting and by pages most often visited. Clicking on any web page in the history list will display the web page. If you are offline, the history allows you to read old content without needing to connect to the web. To alter the maximum number of days for which pages are stored, go to **Tools** → **Internet Options** → **General** → **History**.
- The **Print** button sends the page for printing. If you want to see how the page will look on paper before you print, go to **File** → **Print Preview**. If you want to save a page on your hard drive, go to **File** → **Save As**.

Below the toolbar is the **Address Bar**. This displays the address of the web page being viewed, and is where you enter the address of a website you wish to visit. After entering the address, either press the [RETURN] key or click on the **Go** button. By clicking on the downward-facing arrow on the right side of the address bar, a drop down list will appear of websites you have recently visited. By clicking on a website, it will reappear in the main browser window. The address of a website is also known as the uniform resource locator (URL). URLs are translated into numeric addresses (Internet Protocol, or IP, addresses) using the Domain Name System (DNS), which is a global system of servers that store the location pointers to websites. Once the translation is made by the DNS, the browser can retrieve the file from the web server.

If the web page is larger than can be viewed in the browser window, vertical and horizontal 'scroll bars' will appear down the right-hand side of the screen and across the bottom of the screen, respectively.

At the bottom of the screen is the 'status bar'. This shows the progress of web page downloading and other useful information.

Additional toolbars can be downloaded from the web. For example, the Google Toolbar (*http://www.google.co.uk/contact/tool.html*) gives you access to the Google search engine without needing to go to the Google website. Similarly, the Human Nature Toolbar (human-nature.com) allows you to search resources such as PubMed, Scirus, Encarta, Encyclopedia Britannica and many other sites directly from your Internet Explorer toolbar.

If you want the web page to take up as much of your screen as possible, press [F11] to maximise the browser window and get rid of the menu, address and status bars. Press [F11] again to return to the normal view.

Plug-ins

Although HTML allows the design of attractive web pages that incorporate text and graphics, the designers didn't rest on their laurels but went on to develop 'plug-ins', which are special little programs that work with your web browser to add new functionality. If you come across a website that your browser doesn't know how to handle, you will usually be invited to download the appropriate plug-in from a convenient link. Some common examples are listed below:

- Adobe Acrobat Reader (*http://www.adobe.com/products/acrobat/readstep.html*). Adobe Acrobat allows documents to be distributed, viewed and printed with their original appearance preserved, on any system. The plug-in allows Adobe Acrobat documents available on the web to be viewed within the web browser instead of having to be saved on your hard drive and then opened up in a separate application.
- Macromedia Flash Player (*http://www.macromedia.com/software/flashplayer*) allows you to experience animation and entertainment on the web with Flash, the web standard for vector graphics and animation.
- Macromedia Shockwave Player (*http://www.macromedia.com/software/shockwaveplayer*). Shockwave is the industry standard for delivering high-quality interactive multimedia, graphics and streaming audio on the web.
- RealNetworks' RealPlayer (*http://www.real.com*) lets you play streaming audio, video, animations and multimedia presentations on the web.

- Apple Computer's Quicktime (*http://www.apple.com/quicktime/download*) lets you experience QuickTime animation, music, MIDI, audio, video, and virtual reality panoramas and objects directly in a web page.

If a file cannot be handled either by the browser itself or by a plug-in, it will usually be downloaded.

There are also stand-alone software programs that can enhance your browsing experience:

- Many files are stored and transferred across the Internet in a compressed ('zipped') format, so that they take up less disk space, and consequently take less time to download. 7-Zip is a free program that decompresses these files, making them usable by your computer. Get it at *http://www.7-zip.com*.
- GetRight (*http://www.getright.com*) is a program that accelerates downloads and can recover downloads if errors occur (i.e. can resume downloading). For Linux users, Prozilla (*http://proZilla.genesys.ro*) and Downloader for X (*http://www.krasu.ru/soft/chuchelo*) are similar programs.

Searching the web

Finding web pages may be accomplished in a number of ways, including browsing pages and clicking on links, entering internet addresses into the address bar of the browser and going directly to websites, and using search engines to locate pages on the topic of interest. The sheer number of documents available on the web means that search engines enjoy an important role in allowing users to find the information they are looking for. There are hundreds of search engines, of which Google (*http://www.google.co.uk*) is the most popular at present.

At its simplest, to search for a website requires only the typing of a few descriptive words into a search engine and pressing the [RETURN] key (or clicking on the Google search button) for a list of relevant pages. However, the volume of results may be too great and there are a number of techniques to help reduce the number of results.

- By default, Google will look for pages that include all the words you typed in, even if they do not appear next to each other on the pages found. For example, entering *depression treatment* will return all pages with the words 'depression' and 'treatment', though not necessarily together.
- To search for a phrase, enclose the words in double quote marks. For example, *"depression treatment"* will return all pages in which the exact phrase occurs.
- The search engine may ignore some of your search words. To force the search engine to return only those pages that include a certain word, insert a plus sign before the word. For example, entering *+depression +treatment +fluoxetine* will return only pages that contain all three words.

- To exclude pages that contain a certain word, insert a minus sign (hyphen) in front of that word. For example, *depression treatment -ect* will not return pages which have the abbreviation ECT in them.
- To search for either of two words, use the OR command (note the capital letters). For example, *depression OR dysthmia* will return pages that contain either of these words.
- You can restrict the search to a specific website. For example, *"treatment of depression" site:www.rcpsych.ac.uk* will search the website of the Royal College of Psychiatrists for the specific phrase.

Note that search engines are generally not case sensitive. They may also return results for search terms that are similar to your search words. Some search engines also return 'sponsored links', which have been paid for by advertisers, although they are usually distinguished by, for example, having a different coloured background or being placed on one side of the screen.

As well as searching web pages, Google can also search specifically for images. On the Google home page, select **Images** above the search box and then type in a search term such as *depression*. Instead of web pages, the results show images available on the web. To save an image on your hard drive, move the mouse over the image, click the right mouse button and select **Save Picture As...** Bear in mind that information and images you find on the web may have copyright restrictions on their use.

The Google Company frequently updates the range of services offered, sometimes on a sort of trial (or 'beta') basis. Check out the links above the search box. You will find tools that let you 'Google' the files on your own computer, organise your photo collection, translate foreign languages and hunt for high-quality academic information, to name just a few.

The Google Scholar service (*http://scholar.google.com*) is, at the time of writing, one of these beta services. While not a substitute for Medline, this search service is restricted to scholarly literature, so the quality of information returned should be higher.

Search engines generate their results from massive databases containing information on millions of web pages. Google is an example of a crawler-based search engine. Such search engines repeatedly 'crawl' or 'spider' the web automatically, collecting information on the content of web pages and following links to other sites.

The other main type of search engine is a human-powered directory, such as the Open Directory (*http://dmoz.org*). These depend on humans for their listings. Usually the owner of a website submits a description of the website to the search engine and, if accepted by the editor, the site is added to the search engine.

Many search engines nowadays, such as Yahoo! (*http://uk.yahoo.com*), are a combination of crawler-based and human-powered search engines. There are also search engines that query the databases of other search engines to bring you the most popular results. Examples of such 'meta-search engines' include Mamma (*http://www.mamma.com*) and DogPile (*http://www.dogpile.com*). Ask Jeeves (*http://www.ask.co.uk*) has an extra gimmick in that it encourages you to type in complete sentences in the search box rather than just a few descriptive words.

Bloogz (*http://www.bloogz.com*) is a search engine devoted to locating blogs (web logs, or diaries), which are websites that allow users interactively to share their thoughts with others. For examples, take a look at *http://www.docnotes.net* and *http://www.medpundit.blogspot.com*.

As well as searching for information yourself, you can install software on your computer that will automatically bring updated information from websites to your attention. By subscribing to RSS (Really Simple Syndication) newsfeeds of your choice, you gain access to new or updated information as soon as it is generated. Desktop Sidebar (*http://www.desktopsidebar.com*) is an example of a program that sits on a Windows desktop and displays RSS newsfeeds. A similar program, AmphetaDesk (*http://www.disobey.com/amphetadesk/*), serves Windows, Mac and Linux users.

The problem, as always with the internet, is that anything can be published by anyone. By using careful search techniques you will find sources of reliable and credible information. Some useful websites for psychiatrists are given at the end of the chapter. There are accreditation schemes that evaluate websites, such as the Health On the Net Foundation (*http://www.hon.ch*), but they are not widely used.

Literature searches and citations

In recent years publishers of medical journals have discovered the advantages of distributing their publications rapidly and at low cost using the internet. One example is the *BMJ* site (*http://www.bmj.com*), launched in 1995, which contains the full text of all articles published in the weekly *BMJ* since 1994. In addition, it contains material that is unique to the website. The journals of the Royal College of Psychiatrists are also available online (*http://www.rcpsych.ac.uk/publications/*). The website Free Medical Journals (*http://www.freemedicaljournals.com/*) contains a useful list of other journals available free of charge online.

Access to Medline, the National Library of Medicine's medical literature database, which contains over 11 million abstracts, is available online using the PubMed and Ovid search engines. PubMed is accessible free of charge online (*http://pubmed.gov/*). In contrast, the more powerful Ovid Web Gateway is usually accessible online only through a university network, for which a username and password may be required. An excellent tutorial on using Ovid is available on the Duke University Medical Center Library's website (*http://www.mclibrary.duke.edu/training/ovid/home*). The same principles apply to PubMed.

While it is fairly easy to download references in a form that can be imported into Endnote or other reference management software, it can be even more convenient to search these online databases from *within* your reference management software. James Woolley explains this process in Chapter 8.

Security issues

The browser features that help you can also compromise your security, particularly if other people have access to your computer. You should attend to the following:

- Regularly clear your history folder: **Tools** → **Internet Options** → **Clear History**.
- Regularly delete temporary files generated by your browser: **Tools** → **Internet Options** → **Temporary Files** → **Delete Files**.
- Regularly delete cookies stored on your computer: **Tools** → **Internet Options** → **Temporary Files** → **Delete Cookies**. A cookie is a message given to a web browser by a web server. The browser stores the message in a text file. The message is then sent back to the server each time the browser requests a page from the server. Cookies, although harmless, are used to store things such as passwords for access to websites. If someone shares your computer, they may access to websites that contain personal information.
- Firewalls and antivirus programs are vital for any computer connected to the internet. These are discussed by Mike Madden in Chapter 13.
- Keep your browser up to date. Security vulnerabilities are regularly uncovered in Internet Explorer and are normally corrected by means of a software patch or update. By going to **Tools** → **Windows Update** regularly, you will always have the latest version of the browser.

Telnet

Telnet allows users to log onto computers on the internet and access information resources. Access to Telnet sessions is similar to using the World Wide Web but a Telnet software package is used instead of a browser to access addresses in the form of words or numbers. In contrast to the World Wide Web, Telnet uses text. The lack of graphics and the relative difficulty of using Telnet compared with the World Wide Web have made Telnet increasingly less popular, although it has a place in the toolbox of expert computer users. The similar but more secure Secure Shell (SSH) utility adds encryption to Telnet. The free Putty (*http://www.chiark.greenend.org.uk/~sgtatham/putty/*) program is an excellent Telnet and SSH client.

Usenet newsgroups

Usenet newsgroups are an neglected resource these days. Usenet is a large bulletin board system, on which a wide variety of topics are discussed. The total number of newsgroups totals tens of thousands and with each newsgroup covering one area of interest, there is a newsgroup for nearly every conceivable interest! Once you've found newsgroups of interest, it becomes a strangely addictive pastime.

Newsgroups are electronically held on central computers and users must connect to these to download messages of interest and post their replies, much in the manner of email (see Chapter 11). Combined mail/newsreader software programs are available, such as Outlook Express from Microsoft or the free Thunderbird program (see Chapter 11). Posting and reading messages is similar to composing and reading emails.

The Google search engine maintains an archive of past Usenet discussions. Go to the Google home page (*http://www.google.co.uk*) and click on **Groups**. Much as you would search the World Wide Web, you can also search the Usenet discussion groups. Usenet is particularly useful when you are seeking opinions from other people. For example, search for *bmw cd player problems* and before long you'll know more than most mechanics!

File Transfer Protocol

File Transfer Protocol, or FTP, is a method used to transfer files between computers. Although web browsers can be used, their limited functionality means that most people use specialised software packages such as the excellent and free FileZilla (*http://filezilla.sourceforge.net*). It is mostly used by web designers to upload pages to a server.

A home on the internet

At this point you might be so excited that you want to have your own website! From a technical point of view, this is not difficult. Creating a website involves producing HTML files and then putting them (as well as any graphics or other files) on a web server ('uploading'). There are free programs such as Nvu (*http://www.nvu.com*) which take care of both these tasks and your internet service provider (ISP) has probably already given you a modest amount of space in which to store your creation. If not, a quick Google search for *web hosting* will sort you out.

While not wanting to dampen your enthusiasm, however, there are a few important points to bear in mind.

If you plan on using your website to advertise professional services, you may need to review the relevant professional guidelines on advertising.

If you see your site primarily as a way for people to find and contact you, do remember that disgruntled clients, activists of various stripes and vendors of appendage extension products can use a search engine just as well as your long-lost school friends. Be particularly wary of 'leaking' personal information such as your address or telephone number to websites, forums, blogs and so on.

You need to be aware also that if you run a website, particularly one that accepts content from the public (such as a blog or a forum), you are, in effect, operating as a publisher. David Harris discusses some of the legal implications of this in Chapter 12.

Despite these caveats a personal website can be very useful. It can, for example, act as a sort of 'home' for a distributed project such as a multicentre trial, book or research collaboration. It is easy to add functionality such as file uploads using something like Advanced Transfer Manager (*http://phpatm.free.fr*) or to create a complete forum system like YABB (*http://www.yabbforum.com*), or a collaboratively edited 'wiki' system (*http://www.pmwiki.org*).

These options require a modicum of technical knowledge and some tedious twiddling. You might want to consider outsourcing this by renting a ready-made system such as Basecamp or Backpack from 37 Signals (*http://www.37signals.com*).

Conclusion

The internet is much too large (at least 350 000 000 connected computers as of July 2005 – see *http://www.isc.org*) to cover in a single chapter, or even a single book. However, we do hope that the material in this and other chapters will help get you started. The rest is up to you. In that spirit the following URLs are offered. No responsibility is taken for the content or accuracy of the information contained in these sites, nor should their inclusion be taken as a recommendation.

Useful websites

Organisations

British Medical Association – *http://www.bma.org.uk*
Department of Health – *http://www.dh.gov.uk*
General Medical Council – *http://www.gmc-uk.org*
Modernising Medical Careers – *http://www.mmc.nhs.uk*
National Institute for Clinical Excellence – *http://www.nice.org.uk*
National Institute for Mental Health in England – *http://www.nimhe.org.uk*
Postgraduate Medical Education and Training Board – *http://pmetb.org.uk*
Royal College of Psychiatrists – *http://www.rcpsych.ac.uk*

Journals and bibliographic databases

Advances in Psychiatric Treatment – *http://apt.rcpsych.org*
Archives of General Psychiatry – *http://archpsyc.ama-assn.org*
British Journal of Psychiatry – *http://bjp.rcpsych.org*
BMJ – *http://www.bmj.com*
Psychiatric Bulletin – *http://pb.rcpsych.org*
The Lancet – *http://www.thelancet.com*
Clinical Evidence – *http://www.clinicalevidence.com*
Cochrane Collaboration – *http://www.cochrane.org*
Medline – *http://www.ncbi.nlm.nih.gov/entrez/query.fcgi*

Medico-legal information

HyperGuide Mental Health Act – *http://www.hyperguide.co.uk/mha*
The Institute of Mental Health Act Practitioners – *http://www.markwalton.net*

Pharmacology

British National Formulary – *http://www.bnf.org*
Drugs and Therapeutics Bulletin – *http://www.dtb.org.uk*
Drug Info Zone – *http://www.druginfozone.nhs.uk*
Electronic Medicines Compendium – *http://www.medicines.org.uk*
UK Medicines Information – *http://www.ukmi.nhs.uk*

Psychiatry portals

Medscape – *http://www.medscape.com/psychiatryhome*
Psych Central – *http://www.psychcentral.com*
Psych Direct – *http://www.psychdirect.com*
WHO Guide – *http://www.mentalneurologicalprimarycare.org*

Websites for patients

Royal College of Psychiatrist's mental health information – *http://www.rcpsych.ac.uk/info/index.htm*
BBCi Mental Health – *http://www.bbc.co.uk/health/mental*
National Electronic Library for Mental Health – *http://libraries.nelh.nhs.uk/mentalhealth/*
Patient UK Information Leaflets – *http://www.patient.co.uk*
Talk To Frank (drug addiction) – *http://www.talktofrank.com*
The Good Drugs Guide – *http://www.thegooddrugsguide.com*
OCD Action – *http://www.ocdaction.org.uk*
PTSD Alliance – *http://www.ptsdalliance.org*
Alzheimer's Disease International – *http://www.alz.co.uk*
Anorexia Nervosa and Related Eating Disorders – *http://www.anred.com*
Depression Alliance – *http://www.depressionalliance.org*
Schizophrenia.com – *http://www.schizophrenia.com*

CHAPTER 11

Electronic mail

Bettadapura Ashim and Sindhu Ashim

Email, meaning electronic mail, still comprises the bulk of internet traffic and, according to some commentators, has radically altered the way in which people communicate, including the way that doctors communicate with one another and their patients. How will the increased use of email affect our clinical practice? While we may never go as far as the Americans with consultation by email, it is still an extremely useful tool, with numerous benefits. Email is faster than the post, cheaper and more ecologically friendly. By virtue of being asynchronous (sending and receiving emails can be at different times) email is less interruptive and intrusive than the telephone. Finally, email allows for easy and automatic archiving and searching of correspondence.

Historical background

Over three decades ago Ray Tomlinson sent the first email. In 1971 he was working for a Massachusetts-based company, trying to find a way of allowing users of a computer to leave messages for others on the same machine (like a single-computer version of email). At the same time he was testing a method of sending files to remote computers. It was, ultimately, a matter of bringing these two simple ideas together and in a matter of seconds the '@' symbol was immortalised!

How email works

Emails are text messages, with or without attached files, which are transferred from one computer to the other over the internet. Email is composed and read using email programs or email 'clients' (so-called because they work in a subordinate role to more powerful email 'servers', which are essentially a special type of computer on the internet). Well-known email clients include Microsoft Outlook and Eudora, as well as web-based systems like Hotmail or gMail. Email therefore requires a connection to the internet, either an intermittent dial-up connection or a permanent connection via a local area network (LAN).

After being composed, using an email client, the email is either sent immediately or kept in the 'outbox' until the sender's computer is next connected to the internet. It is then transferred (after the sender proves his or her identity) to an email server. Somewhat confusingly, the term server refers to both the server computer itself (the hardware) and the software that runs on it. This email server software receives the message and passes it on to the recipient's email server (typically that owned by the recipient's internet service provider), where it will remain until the recipient (via an email client) checks his or her account. After another identity check, the email is then transferred, or 'downloaded', to the recipient's computer. Figure 11.1 outlines the process.

There are three main types of standard email servers: SMTP (Simple Mail Transfer Protocol), IMAP (Internet Mail Access Protocol) and POP3 (Post Office Protocol, version 3). SMTP deals with outgoing email and email in transit, whereas IMAP and POP3 deal with incoming email.

In the past, if, for some reason, you were unable to use the SMTP server of your own organisation, you could have submitted your email to any SMTP server for onward delivery. Similarly, SMTP servers passed mail onto one another for relaying. Such 'open relays' were often exploited by spammers (senders of unsolicited emails; spam is discussed below) as a way of

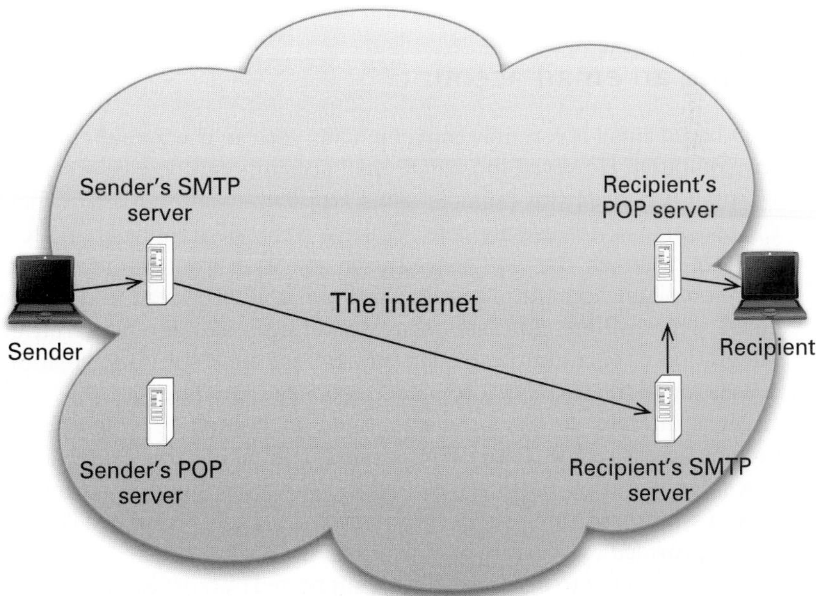

Fig. 11.1 How email works.

hiding their identities. As a result, modern SMTP servers tend to be rather selective about those from whom they accept email. If the SMTP server belongs to the same organisation that provides your current internet connection, then your mail will be accepted (usually) without question. If, however, your try to access your 'home' SMTP server via your work network or vice versa, you may need to configure your mail client to prove your identity in some way, to 'authenticate' the email. This option will typically be found under 'SMTP configuration' or similar (this is discussed in detail below).

The POP protocol allows email clients to authenticate and then download emails for a particular user on the POP server (delivered by the SMTP server). By default the emails are then deleted from the POP server, though this behaviour can usually be changed.

Email began as a text-only medium but more recently any kind of file can be sent with (attached to) an email. Attachments are governed by the MIME (Multipurpose Internet Mail Extensions) protocol, which is usually made simple for the end-user.

This (highly simplified) model of email technology is complicated slightly by so-called webmail systems such as Hotmail from MSN or gMail from Google. These work in the same way as above except for the last step, where the recipient accesses mail via POP email. Web-based email is accessed instead via a web browser, such as Internet Explorer or Firefox. Instead of transferring the email to the email client on the recipient's computer, it is kept on the server and displayed to the recipient as a web page. Emails are retrieved by visiting the email provider's site and entering a username and password.

Selecting an email account

Web-based email is certainly convenient, as you can check your email from any computer. However, most POP mail accounts can now be accessed as webmail if desired (for example using *http://www.mail2web.com*), whereas the converse is not usually true. While a webmail account is fine for an internet beginner, the experienced user will soon want the features of a POP-compliant account. These include the ability to read and compose email while offline, for later sending, filing email for later retrieval, integration of email into calendar and address book software, creation of aliases for addresses, and automated tools like spam filters.

Most internet service providers, such as Demon or Freeserve, also provide access to SMTP and POP servers, and taking this route certainly eases configuration hassles (see above). However, there is no technical reason why these three services (internet access, POP and SMTP) could not be provided by separate organisations.

IMAP is similar to POP email and is supported by most email clients, but the messages are retained on the server even after they have been checked.

This offers more flexibility, as messages can be accessed from any computer. IMAP is usually the province of the 'power user' of email.

Another decision facing a newcomer to email is whether to use a free or a paid-for service. You are advised to bear in mind that 'you get what you pay for'. In practical terms the annual fee for a reliable, reputable, professional POP email provider is negligible compared with the humiliation of having your incisive letter to the *BMJ* cited as being from *joe99@hotpants.com*!

Many hospitals and trusts have their own email account, which is ideal for clinical and professional use. These may or may not be accessible outside the workplace as they are usually POP or IMAP accounts. A disadvantage for trainees who move hospitals is that this email address cannot follow them. The new NHSmail initiative (*http://www.nhs.net*) is intended to address this problem. NHSmail accounts currently offer 64 megabytes of storage, are secure and can be accessed from any computer connected to the internet. Megabytes (MB) are discussed in Chapter 1, but, as an example, a typical snapshot from a modest digital camera would be about 1 MB in size.

Choosing an email client

If you follow the advice above and choose a POP or IMAP account, then you can rest assured that you can access your email with any modern email client.

Windows computers come with an email client called Outlook Express. There have, however, been some security concerns with this program and the reader may be advised to look elsewhere.

Thunderbird (available to download at *http://www.mozilla.org/products/thunderbird/*) is a companion to the Firefox browser mentioned in Chapter 10 and is a free choice (in every sense). Eudora (*http://www.eudora.com*) comes in both advertising-supported and paid versions. Commercial alternatives include Pocomail (*http://www.pocosystems.com/home/index.php*) and The Bat! (*http://www.ritlabs.com/en/products/thebat/*). (See Chapter 1 for details on how to install software.)

Both Eudora and Thunderbird come in versions for Windows and Mac and Thunderbird in addition is available for Linux. For that reason, and because it is a free download, we will use Thunderbird in the example that follows, although the configuration and use of other clients differ only in minor details.

Configuring your email client

To configure your email client you will have to enter your name, email address, the addresses of your chosen POP and SMTP servers and any passwords. These will be available from your internet service provider,

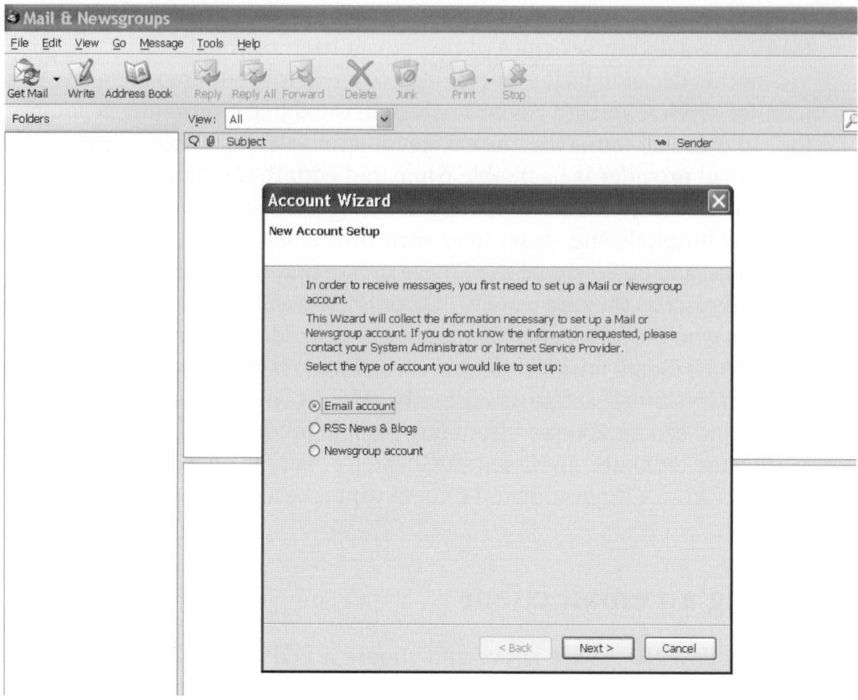

Fig. 11.2 Account wizard.

on the website of your chosen provider or in the printed material that you received.

Most email clients, when started for the first time, offer a series of screens provided by as a 'wizard' as an easy way to configure an account (Fig. 11.2). You then just put the information in the boxes and click **Next**.

The first couple of screens merely ask you to confirm that you want to set up an email account and ask for your name and email address. The hard questions concerning your incoming (POP) and outgoing (SMTP) servers come in the next screen (Fig. 11.3).

The wizard will end with a helpful summary of the information you entered (Fig. 11.4) before going ahead and implementing your instructions.

Suppose you mess up the first time you try to create an account or you want to add a second account (multiple email accounts are both possible and very useful). The same configuration information can be entered at a later stage. In most clients this is achieved by a menu option such as **Tools → Account Settings** (Fig. 11.5). The relevant section may also lurk under menu items such as **Preferences** or **Options**. In Thunderbird, clicking the **Add Account** button will restart the wizard. More advanced settings (such as server authentication and encryption) can also be set here.

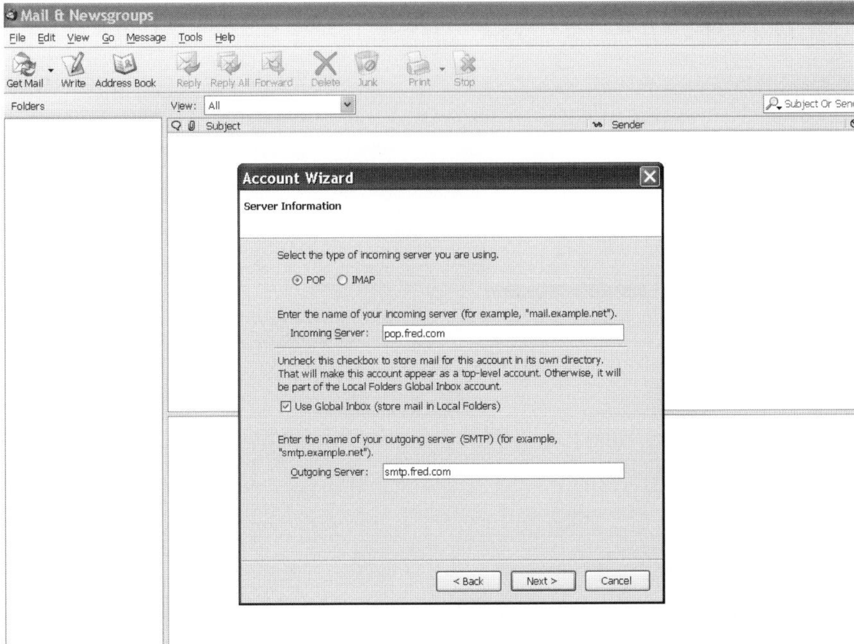

Fig. 11.3 Setting the server configuration in the account wizard.

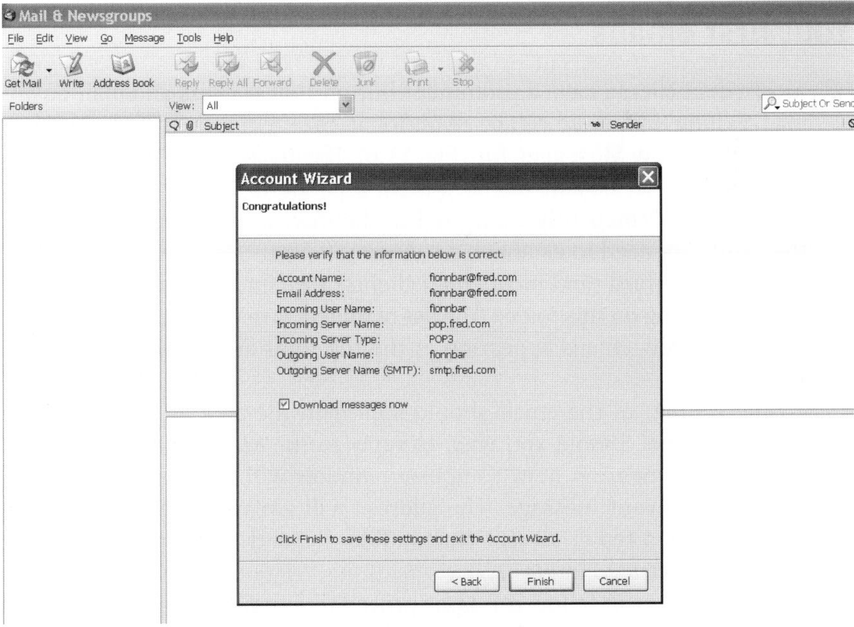

Fig. 11.4 Configuration summary in the account wizard.

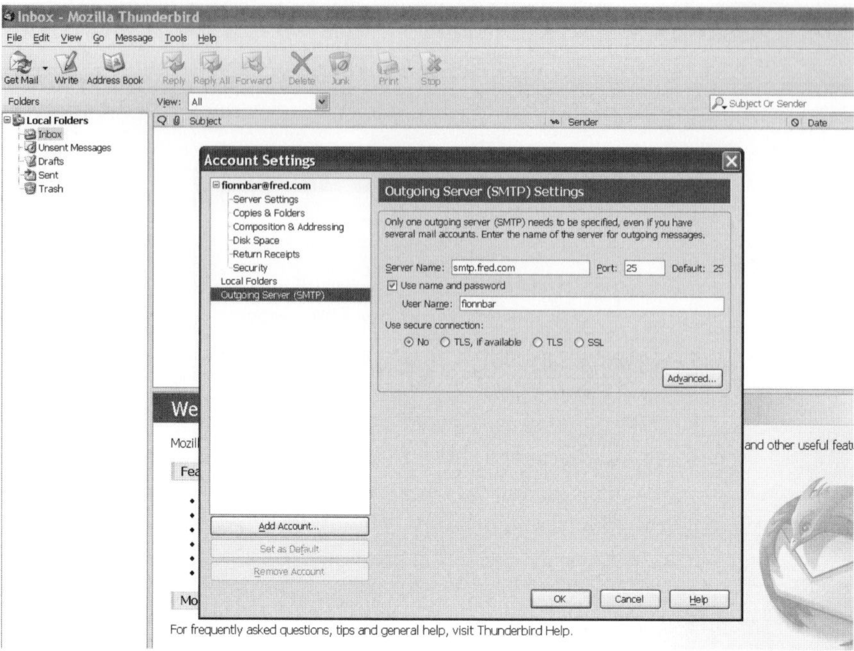

Fig. 11.5 The Account Settings screen.

Your first emails

Most email clients have a prominent button that triggers an email download. Failing that, there will be an option in the menus; in Thunderbird it is **File → Get New Messages for** (Fig. 11.6). If you have more than one email account you may be able to check them separately, which can be useful. If you are not permanently connected to the internet (i.e. you use dial-up), then you may need to establish a connection first.

In Thunderbird (and most email clients) new emails arrive in the *Inbox* folder. Clicking on this folder (the list of folders is on the left) should result in a list of new emails appearing in the top right area of your client (see Fig. 11.7).

The content of the email should appear in the area under this in the 'preview' pane. Should you wish to reply to the email, click **Message → Reply** in the menu. A new 'composer' window will spring open, in which you can type your message. The address will already have been filled in (since this is a reply) so just choose **File → Send Now** or **File → Send Later**, as illustrated in Fig. 11.8.

For a new email follow the same procedure but fill in the email address yourself. Addresses can also be found in the address book (click on the **Address Book** icon shown in Fig. 11.7).

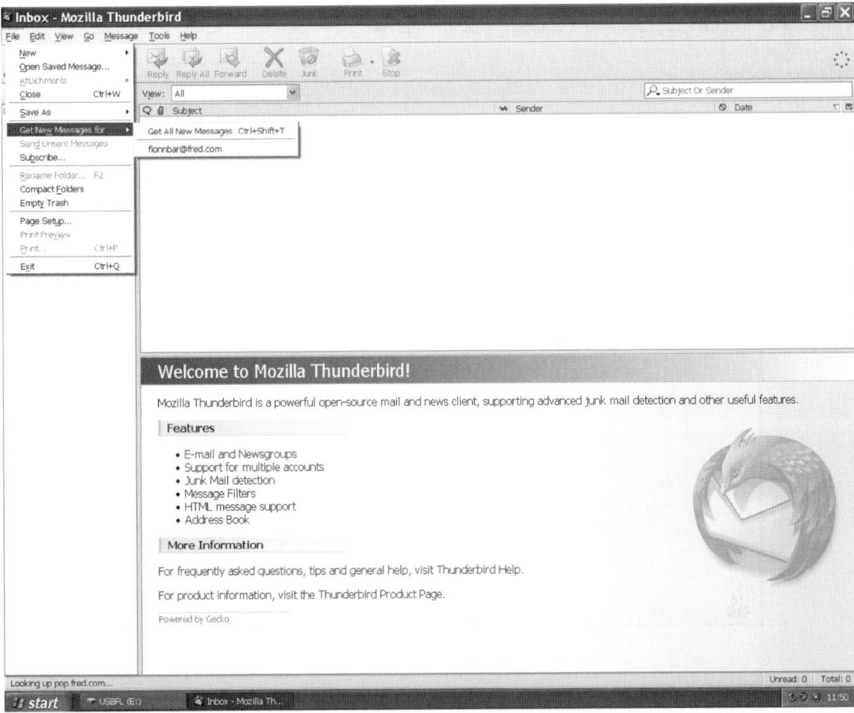

Fig. 11.6 Checking mail.

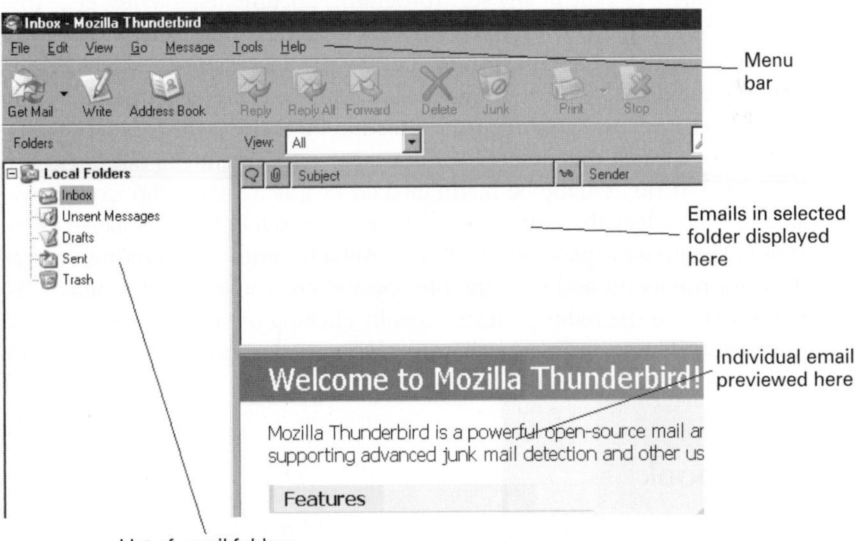

Fig. 11.7 The main screen.

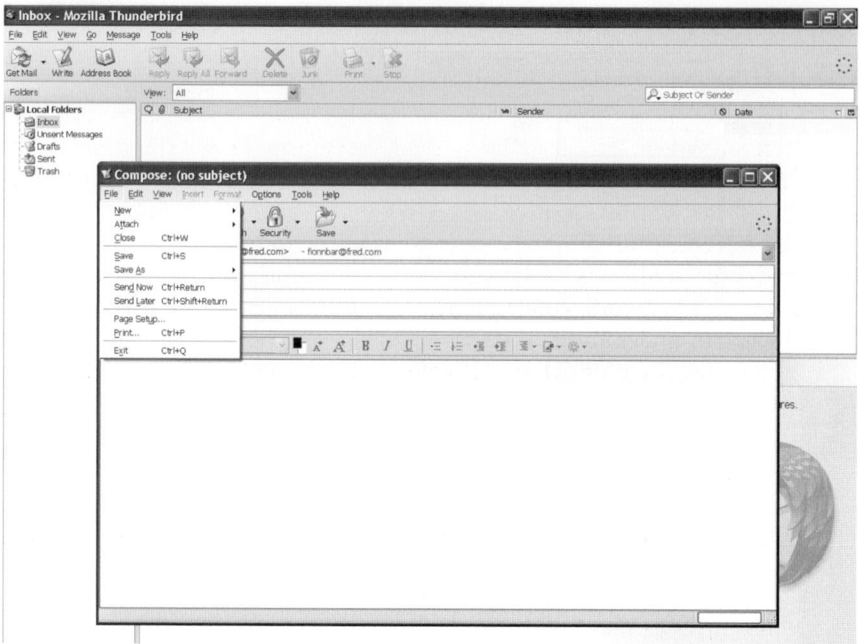

Fig. 11.8 Sending email.

Attachments

An attachment is a file of any sort (programs, documents, movies, etc.) that is sent along with an email. To attach a file to an outgoing email in Thunderbird click on the paperclip icon in the compose window (or select **File → Attach**) and navigate through the file system (see Chapter 1) to the file you want. Click on it and confirm your selection by clicking the **Open** button.

Besides the fact that an email with a large attachment can take an age to download, it can usually be distinguished by a little paperclip icon to one side. If you select the email, you will see the attachment displayed as an icon in the preview pane. Select **File → Attachments → Filename → Save As** from the menu and save the file somewhere you can find it again. Try not to get into the habit of automatically clicking on attachments to open them immediately and always beware that not all attachments are friendly – some may contain viruses (see below).

Address book

Thunderbird, like most email clients, has an address book. Addresses from received emails can be easily added to the address book by right clicking ([CTRL] click on a Mac) on the address in the preview pane.

Sorting your email

By default most email clients come with *Inbox, Outbox, Sent* and *Draft* folders. You will probably want to create more folders as your email accumulates. To do this in Thunderbird use **File → New → Folder**. Folders can have subfolders and so on but don't overdo this. Your computer can search all your emails for keywords (**Edit → Find → Search Messages**), so this represents an alternative to obsessive filing.

Another option is to delegate the filing to the computer by setting up 'rules' or filters for incoming email. The relevant function in Thunderbird is accessed under **Tools → Message Filters**. Of course, this can lead to the interesting situation where all your email is neatly organised but never read!

Some guidelines for filtering

- Clarify your information priorities. What are the main categories of information that you will use again and again?
- Try and be consistent between your PC folders, email folders and personal organiser.
- Don't be afraid to file a single email in several folders. Many people like to retain one copy of the non-trash email in the *In* folder since they can often remember roughly when an email was received.
- If your email is linked to a wider office system, perhaps you can add some relevant keyword before you file.
- Set criteria for what you want to file and save. Why keep email when you can use your intranet or the internet to retrieve key information or documents?
- Do some occasional cleansing. You may have a system that prompts regularly to decide which messages that are three months old or more, for example, you want to keep.

Auto-responding

An advantage of using an email client is the ability to set up an automatic response for when you are away from your desk, say when you go home in the evening or when you are away for a few weeks on vacation. Auto-responding has peculiar problems and not all email providers allow you to configure an auto-response. The reason is that if several people have auto-response turned on, they will keep bouncing messgaes to each other and can crash servers! Auto-responders can also interact unpredictably with mailing lists. You are advised therefore to seek the guidance of your email provider or information technology support before implementing this feature.

Forwarding

Most email clients make it very easy, perhaps too easy, to forward the currently selected message. Although this is convenient for group working, it has drawbacks and can contribute to 'information overload'. Think also about whether the original sender would want the email forwarded.

Mailing lists

Most email clients allow you to set up small mailing lists, which facilitate efficient communication with multiple recipients. Larger mailing lists are hosted on servers and make use of special software. Many publicly accessible mailing lists can be found at *http://www.lsoft.com/lists/listref.html*. Mailing lists may also be provided by your organisation. For example, there may be a mailing list for all consultants in the hospital.

Hazards of email

Spam

Spam is unsolicited commercial or 'junk' email sent to a very large number of users at once. The internet holds millions of email addresses and provides an irresistible temptation for salespeople. Because the net is so vast and mailing is so cheap (no postage fees!) there is no reason for spammers to narrow down their mailing lists. So your child receives the same advertisement for Viagra as the pensioner in another part of the world. AOL recently said that a third of their network capacity was consumed by spam.

Many spam emails advertise illegal products, promote fraudulent schemes or carry hazardous content such as obscene material or viruses as attachments. For these reasons it is essential to protect your email address and keep it private. Just as you would not give out your home address to strangers, be cautious when giving out your email address in chat rooms, forums, online contests and surveys. A popular free program to block spam is Spambutcher, which is downloadable at *http://www.spambutcher.com*.

Never reply to spam email. If an email asks you to 'unsubscribe' by following a link or by replying with 'unsubscribe' in the subject box, ignore it as it is probably just a ploy to get you to confirm your email address as active and open for more spam.

Avoid forwarding chain letters or petitions. Mass mailings like this constitute spam in themselves and the lists of addresses on them are often used by spammers.

Trojans, viruses and worms

Mike Madden deals with this bestiary of malicious software in Chapter 13. Here we will only touch on the issues that relate to email.

Never open an email attachment from a stranger. Even if an email is from someone you know you may still be at risk since some viruses harvest email addresses from the addresses books of infected computers. Another common ploy is to disguise malicious emails as routine 'bounced' email error messages.

Emails with an attachment such as *.pif* or *.exe* or *.scr* are even more likely to be malicious code. Delete them straight away without opening them.

The crucial thing to remember is that it is not wise to download or open an attachment unless you are expecting to receive a file.

Antivirus software is essential. There are several commercial products such as Norton and McAfee which cost around £50 to buy and £30 per year to receive updates. Antivirus software has to be updated frequently as newer viruses are created every day. Updates are usually downloadable from the web. Alternatively, free antivirus software is available. Grisoft's AVG is one of the most popular and can be downloaded from *http://free.grisoft.com/freeweb.php/doc/2/lng/us/tpl/v5*.

Lost productivity

Many of us start the day by checking our email, preferably with a cup of coffee in hand. A common pattern is then to keep on working with the email client open in the background. It may even be set to alert us with a ping when a new email arrives. This may not be the most efficient pattern, however. Constant interruptions get in the way of focusing on demanding tasks. A day spent dealing with urgent but unimportant emails is a day wasted. Setting aside a number of periods during the day to deal with email might be a more productive use of time.

The judicious use of mailing lists, both formal and ad hoc, as described above, can also boost productivity.

It has been our experience that much of the email arriving in a typical National Health Service account is, if not formally spam, at least highly irrelevant. A little time spent politely requesting to be removed from these email circulars might be a good investment. Alternatively it might be possible to filter these emails off and file them in a separate folder, where they can be scanned at leisure.

Many experienced email users have a 'disposable' account for posting on web pages or mailing lists (from where it can be harvested by spammers) and a 'serious' address that is handed out only to trusted contacts. Free, web-based accounts are good for the former.

There are several good sources of information on email productivity on the internet (e.g. *http://www.43folders.com/2005/02/15/five-fast-email-productivity-tips/*).

Netiquette

There is no universally agreed set of rules governing email. However, the following suggestions incorporate general principles of basic courtesy and respect.

- Do not spam or indulge in excessive forwarding. It clutters up servers and inboxes and can be very annoying. Do not forward information about other people without their consent.
- Do not send large attachments; the recipient's account may not have the space. It is best to send text in the body of the email rather than as an attachment if possible.
- Keep messages brief and format them for easy reading. Delete irrelevant text, especially if email has been back and forth several times using the 'reply' option. It may, however, be appropriate to leave the text in if there is a risk of losing the thread of communication.
- Recently it has become possible to use, for example, bold, underlined text in emails. Try to avoid the temptation to use this fancy (so-called rich text or HTML) formatting in your emails. This may not be readable by some computers or email programs and may cause security problems. There will probably be an item under **Options** that will let you turn this off.
- Make use of the subject line to summarise the message.
- Use the 'BCC' field (to send a 'blind' copy) when sending email to multiple recipients to avoid spammers exploiting and harvesting email addresses.
- Do not forward chain emails (emails requesting you to forward them to other users), including virus warnings and petitions for good causes. Simply delete them. Most organisations have policies against forwarding chain emails as it can clog networks and waste disk space.
- Do not 'flame' or send abusive, harassing or threatening emails. If you find yourself writing a nasty email, do not send it. Save it and come back after a while. Be careful when using humour and sarcasm: it can easily be misinterpreted without the advantages of face-to-face communication.
- Email is not confidential. If you have a professional email account through your hospital or organisation, the content may be screened. Laws governing copyright, defamation, discrimination and other forms of written communication also apply to email. Beware of illegal activities such as sending illegal adult material or incitement to violence (see Chapter 12).
- Allow time for responding to emails. Although it is possible to mark an email as 'urgent' or 'high priority', you should use this sparingly, if at all.

Email in the National Health Service

Clinical use

Email, when encrypted, can offer a high degree of security, but care by users is still required. For example, if emails are sent to a non-encrypted email account such as Hotmail the security is lost. See Chapters 12 and 13 for a fuller treatment of the legal and security issues involved in sending patient information by email. Until such problems have been overcome, you are advised to consult the information technology department of your organisation before starting down the road of integrating email into clinical practice.

Professional use

Email facilitates effective communication with large numbers of colleagues about professional matters such as meetings. Opinion polls and surveys can also be conducted in a fraction of the time they would take by post.

Trips to libraries, queues for photocopying machines, waiting for borrowed journals – all these are things of the past. It is easy to keep track of the ever-growing medical literature by setting up email alerts through various library resources, such as the National electronic Library for Health (*http://www.nelh.nhs.uk*).

Another use of email alerts is for job hunting. The *BMJ*'s classified edition can be customised to send email alerts about jobs that match specified requirements.

Administrative uses

Email can be used for administrative purposes such as arranging out-patient appointments, reporting selected test results, completing medical forms and writing prescriptions.

Email communication with patients

'Clinician–patient email' is communication with patients within a contractual relationship, where the healthcare provider takes explicit responsibility for patients' care. 'Clinician–patient email' is uncommon in the UK but is gaining popularity in the United States. There are no official guidelines setting out safeguards for communication between clinicians and patients and individual trusts are expected to develop their own. Guidelines published by the American Medical Informatics Association on the clinical use of email with patients is perhaps the most comprehensive and best available (see Further reading).

Electronic communication has the potential to improve efficiency and patient satisfaction when used to complement personal contact between clinician and patient. There are some anecdotal and survey data that show patients are more satisfied when they have email access to their providers (see Further reading). Patients may feel pressured in a time-limited clinic setting, whereas email can offer a very non-threatening platform. It is particularly useful for certain niche populations, such as those requiring monitoring of chronic conditions.

There are risks and benefits of email communication with patients. Some suggestions for successful implementation are as follows:

- The introduction of clinician–patient email needs to be approved of and supported by the healthcare provider involved.
- There need to be clear policies governing informed consent to email correspondence, data protection, privacy issues, delay in response, holiday cover arrangements, and so on.
- Resources need to be allocated to support this mode of working.
- Email must be a supplement to, and not a replacement for, face-to-face contact, particularly with the 'electronically disenfranchised'.

In this chapter we have struck some cautionary notes. Despite these caveats the use of email within healthcare is set to increase and continue to change our practice as doctors and professionals.

Further reading

Kane, B. & Sands, D. Z. (1998) Guidelines for the clinical use of electronic mail with patients. *Journal of the American Medical Informatics Association*, **5**, 104–111.

Sands, D. Z. (1999) Electronic patient-centred communication: managing risks, managing opportunities, managing care. *American Journal of Managed Care*, **5**, 1569–1571.

CHAPTER 12

Legal issues pertaining to the use of information technology within psychiatry

David Harris

When first asked to write this chapter I was concerned that the field was too narrow and esoteric. On further investigation, however, I found that there was no shortage of material. Information technology (IT) is already pervasive in society and has transformed itself from being an optional tool to a part of the fabric of many professions, including psychiatry and medicine. The risks faced by psychiatrists are generally those faced by other professionals with relatively few profession-specific variations thrown in. In an ever more litigious and rule-bound society it is important to be aware of these risks.

The chapter is divided into two sections. The first deals with civil matters (for example disputes between individuals) and the second with criminal matters (where the state prosecutes and imposes sanctions).

Civil matters

Confidentiality

Confidentiality is a matter of vital importance to psychiatrists and their patients, and this view is reflected in both case and statute law. The only grounds for breaching patient confidentiality generally involve risk to specific third parties or to the community. IT systems, however, have the potential for serious confidentiality breaches. Many of these problems are being swept aside by a government striving to contain costs and enhance the abilities of law enforcement and security agencies.

New proposals for national electronic patient record systems may give professionals from external agencies access to clinical data held on National Health Service (NHS) computers (see Chapter 14). While promising better communication between agencies and a more seamless service, there are three main disadvantages:

- It may give access to highly sensitive patient information to staff with no real 'need to know'.

- Such a complex system is difficult to secure against intruders or 'crackers' (criminal hackers).
- From a professional perspective, there is also the worrying possibility that the doctor who gathered and recorded the leaked information could be held responsible for any resulting breaches in confidentiality.

The challenge, therefore, is to get the benefits of such systems while eliminating, or at least mitigating, the risks. This will require an open and honest discussion, something that has, to date, been lacking.

Emails and websites

Email is inherently insecure. The technical underpinnings of internet email are such that interception cannot easily be detected or prevented. Mail can also be forwarded against the wishes of the original sender. This problem is not unique to electronic communication but the ease and pseudo-intimacy of email as compared with letters may lead the parties into inappropriate disclosures. Consider the following email:

> From: Dr.M.Barratt@myhealthtrust.nhs.uk
> To: P.Mckay@myhealthtrust.nhs.uk
> Subject: John Gray - NHS number XXX00
>
> Peter,
>
> Mr Gray's new complaint against me is that it I was negligent in his treatment and that as a result he has been unable to obtain further work as a bricklayer. He also complains that he is now shunned in the village of Little Eden in Sussex as a result of the failed treatment.
>
> I remain confident in my diagnosis that he has post-traumatic stress and that his sexual and relationship problems do stem from his employment as we discussed. Although not strictly relevant to this issue, I have attached copies of my notes of his last two sessions in case they are useful to you...

This would probably represent the flavour of many emails circulated by health professionals and it violates privacy principles in several ways, including the Caldicott principles that we will discuss later.

If, as a result of previous conversations, the recipient will know who is being talked about, then it might be better simply to refer to 'the JG issue' or 'the PTS patient' or even 'ref XXX00'. Similarly, the inclusion of the patient's address and profession as well as the peripheral notes would be difficult to justify.

An even more acute danger is represented by the latest trend in web publishing, 'blogging' (web logging – see Chapter 10). These online diaries are used as a form of self-expression and communication by many people, doctors included. The danger is that, seduced by the medium, the doctor will inadvertently breach Caldicott principles. No such examples have yet come to light but it is probably only a matter of time.

System security

Accidental loss, theft, repair and the disposal of old computers and storage media (floppies and CDs) can leave your patient's information in the hands of a stranger. Even trusted staff (e.g. a secretary) can abuse their position by accessing data that they have no reason or right to see. Some viruses can even email interesting documents back to their creators. What liability might a doctor face in these situations?

It is not beyond the bounds of possibility that the doctor would suffer the double misfortune of first being a victim of computer crime and then being held liable for professional misconduct as a result. While this might seem a little unfair, the reason (as Mike Madden will explain in Chapter 13) is that there are relatively simple ways to protect sensitive information, such as using file and folder encryption. This solution is ideal for those with laptops and I would regard it as mandatory if a hard drive or removable drive contains patient data. To my knowledge no doctor has yet been held liable for such failures but this is a real possibility for the future.

Non-statutory controls: the Caldicott principles

The use of personal information in the UK is guided by a series of rules known as the Caldicott principles. Since they lack a statutory basis, failure to follow these principles is not unlawful; however, they form an integral part of best clinical practice and failure to follow them would constitute a *prima facie* argument for liability in the event of a claim against a doctor for negligence. The principles are briefly described below.

1 *Justify the purpose(s)*. Every proposed use or transfer of personally identifiable information within or from an organisation should be clearly defined and scrutinised, with continuing uses regularly reviewed by that organisation's 'Caldicott guardian'.
2 *Don't use personally identifiable information unless it is absolutely necessary*. Such information should not be used unless there is no alternative.
3 *Use the minimum necessary personally identifiable information*. Where use of personally identifiable information is considered to be essential, each individual item of information should be justified, with the aim of reducing identifiability.
4 *Access to personally identifiable information should be on a strict 'need to know' basis*. Only those individuals who need access to personally identifiable information should have access to it, and they should have access only to the information items they need to see for a specific purpose.
5 *Everyone should be aware of their responsibilities*. Action should be taken to ensure that those handling personally identifiable information, both practitioner and non-practitioner staff, are aware of their responsibilities and obligations to respect an individual's confidentiality.
6 *Understand and comply with the law*. Every use of personally identifiable information must be lawful. Each organisation must identify a Caldicott

guardian responsible for ensuring that the organisation complies with legal requirements.

Clinical implications of Caldicott

While most NHS organisations have well-developed Caldicott systems (and you are advised to seek these out), it is important to realise that, when operating in private practice, the responsibility for compliance falls on the individual doctor (as ultimately it does when the doctor is employed by the NHS). What follows, then, is a discussion of the most prominent issues in the light of Caldicott.

Legal controls

The Caldicott principles are an addition to, not a substitute for, the legal protections of confidentiality. These legal protections arise from both statute law (i.e. acts passed by Parliament) and common law, and apply to confidentiality generally, not just in the medical context.

The main statute governing data is the Data Protection Act 1998 (see below). This controls both electronic and paper records. Also relevant are such miscellaneous provisions as the Road Traffic Act, the Health and Safety at Work Act and the notifiable disease laws.

Thus far we have spoken rather loosely of 'confidentiality' without providing the legal meaning. Let me correct that. The root of the legal obligation of confidentiality is that there is a relationship between the utterer of the confidence and its recipient. Some, but by no means all, relationships give rise to a duty to protect certain types of information. To be protected by the law of confidentiality the information need not have been kept secret but it should not be in the public domain and it should ordinarily be difficult to find. It should also be of such a nature that its release would be damaging to the owner. Given its sensitivity, personal medical data fall squarely into this category. An obligation of confidentiality will be imposed by the courts on all those who handle such data if they attempt to use it beyond the purpose for which it was revealed. By contrast, the statutes do not talk of confidential information but rather personal data, which provides for a broader range of protected material.

The Data Protection Act

There are eight underlying principles to the Act that govern the use of personal data. The principles state that personal data should be:

1 fairly and lawfully processed
2 processed for limited purposes
3 adequate, relevant and not excessive for the purpose for which they were collected
4 kept in a secure manner
5 accurate

6 not kept longer than necessary for the purpose
7 processed according to the rights of the data subject
8 not transferred to countries with an inadequate data protection regime.

Some personal data are more sensitive than others – for example, trade union membership, political affiliation, diseases, sexual orientation or other medical information – and such data have more rigorous protection. In the case of sensitive personal data, schedules to the Act impose requirements on using, or 'processing' in the language of the Act, the data. With some exceptions that we will discuss later, data are to be used with the consent of the patient, for his or her benefit or for the purposes of legal action or where using it is necessary for medical purposes. Exceptions exist for monitoring purposes and research that doesn't immediately benefit the patient but which is in the wider public interest.

Fair processing of information

The first data protection principle has some implications for the medical profession. The patient should be told who is processing the data (e.g. an NHS trust or a private practice), what the data are and for what purpose they are being used. This does not necessarily involve giving long, detailed descriptions but giving just enough information to alert the patient to potential privacy risks and so allow him or her to take advice or object, for example where information to be gathered is optional or if the patient wants to prevent others getting it. It may be appropriate to tell the patient about not just the clinical data but also related information if this is relevant, such as family relationships and employment. However, a doctor is not required to show the patient large amounts of information he or she already knows.

Perhaps one of the most important exceptions relevant to mental health professionals is the exception in section 29 of the Data Protection Act: this allows the use or processing of data for the prevention or detection of crime or the prosecution of offenders. In these circumstances, it is lawful to disclose personal information without informing the 'data subject' (i.e. the patient) or to process such data without informing him or her. For example, if an offender made confessions during a clinical session it would be lawful to disclose that confession together with the relevant portions (and *only* the relevant portions) of the patient's medical records to the police.

Medical data and confidentiality: the exceptions

We've discussed the general scope of confidentiality above, but some exceptions have long been recognised in relation to medical data. For example, communicable diseases have long been subject to a reporting requirement. Likewise, section 60 of the Health and Social Care Act 2001 empowers the Secretary of State to use patient-identifiable information without the consent of patients and overriding any normal duty of confidence, where it is deemed necessary for the support of NHS activity. Similarly, when there is an overriding duty to the public, a legal compulsion arises to disclose information, or if the patient has consented, then confidential information can be released. Inevitably this involves careful assessment of whether the rights of the public outweigh those of the patient and that is something for which there is no general guidance, since it will depend on the individual facts of the case.

Objecting to data use

Section 10 of the Data Protection Act provides a remedy for the data subject to object to the use of data. The section says:

'(1) Subject to subsection (2), an individual is entitled at any time by notice in writing to a data controller to require the data controller at the end of such period as is reasonable in the circumstances to cease, or not to begin, processing, or processing for a specified purpose or in a specified manner, any personal data in respect of which he is the data subject, on the ground that, for specified reasons –

(a) the processing of those data or their processing for that purpose or in that manner is causing or is likely to cause substantial damage or substantial distress to him or to another, and

(b) that damage or distress is or would be unwarranted.'

Thus objections need to be in writing and the grounds of justification are the distress the processing would cause the data subject. It is necessary to act within 21 days of such a notice. Doctors in receipt of such a notice of objection do not necessarily have to comply with it: they may, for example, be under a legal obligation to process the data; a research exception may be applicable; the data subject may have previously consented; or it may be in the data subject's vital interests that the processing happens.

Human rights legislation

The European Convention on Human Rights (ECHR), as embedded in English law by the Human Rights Act 1988, has an important role in medical confidentiality. Article 8 states that 'Everyone has a right to respect for his private and family life, his home and his correspondence'. Case law on the ECHR and Human Rights Act confirms that Article 8 applies to medical data.

In the case of *Z* v. *Finland* the court said that 'medical data, is of fundamental importance to a person's enjoyment of his or her right to respect for private and family life'. On the facts of the case it was said the Finnish authorities were entitled to reveal the person's medical data in a criminal case since the right was subject to two saving qualifications: the prevention of crime and the protection of the rights of others. However, there was still a violation of her right to confidentiality when her identity was revealed. It's clear, then, that human rights do not provide absolute rights to patients: it is a careful balance of the needs of the patient and society.

Online liability

The burden of all professionals, be they lawyers or psychiatrists, is to be plagued by requests for free help and advice; those who yield to such requests on the internet, as elsewhere, run the risk of incurring professional liability.

Online negligence

No medical professional needs telling about the dangers of negligence attached to the diagnosis and treatment of patients. When strangers present with symptoms in a web forum the dangers are compounded. An informal, quasi-social environment may lull doctors into reducing the standards applied from those that they would enforce in a more formal clinical setting. For example, it may be difficult to take a proper medical history in a public forum. Professional standards will, none the less, be applied in undiluted form by any court if litigation results from negligence: anything done online will be subject to the same standards of professionalism that would be applied offline.

At law, an accusation of negligence is assessed by asking whether there was a relationship of proximity between the parties. If there was, then the question asked is whether a duty of care was breached by the acts done and whether the damage that was caused was reasonably foreseeable.

In a conventional clinical setting there is unlikely to be much doubt that a duty of care is owed by a psychiatrist to a patient: the doctor must be diligent to the standards of the profession. In an informal online context, however, it could be argued that the principle that 'you get what you pay for' (i.e. not very much) applies and there is little basis for complaint.

At one time this was the judicial attitude: Lord Denning once said that there was no liability for an off-the-cuff remark made on the phone. Updated for the internet this would seem to imply that some forms of communication, such as 'chat' or 'instant messaging', might be exempt.

Unfortunately, subsequent case law has imposed liability where advice was given in a social situation. In one case a woman obtained the assistance of a knowledgeable friend when buying a car that later turned out to be defective. The adviser was held liable, despite not charging for his advice. This was largely because he assumed liability for his advice by discouraging her from obtaining the advice of a qualified mechanic. It may well be that a court would say that it was reasonable to assume that a person would rely on the advice of a professional even when casually given. It may also be that there would be no liability at all or that damages would be reduced, perhaps by a substantial amount, because the recipient of the advice should have confirmed it with his or her own doctor and that by not doing so was contributorily negligent.

Many medical sites will contain a disclaimer to the effect that no one should rely on advice without seeking the opinion of their own doctor. In the light of the above discussion, this would seem to be both understandable and probably effective. None the less, the entire subject of disclaimers and their effectiveness remains a grey area for lawyers.

On those occasions when the author is asked for free legal advice at parties, he always advises his interlocutors to speak to their own lawyer before doing anything. The reader may wish to do likewise.

Record-keeping

When the basis of any accusation against a doctor is his or her online conduct, then, where possible, a record of that conduct should be kept, for example by archiving emails or other messages. It may be felt that by deleting embarrassing communications there is no 'smoking gun'. However, if this is done, then the only evidence left may be that of the accuser, who is likely to have kept records.

Making records may not always be possible either technically or practically, but where facilities exist they should be used. Many chat and instant messaging programs have a logging feature that could be used to create a transcript. Search engines such as Google automatically store postings to newsgroups and forums, which can later be searched.

Many people try to preserve records for at least six years (the duration of the Statute of Limitations, after which one cannot normally be sued) but in some cases this may cause a problem if the accusation is one of those not subject to the statute.

Jurisdiction

One of the other primary issues with the internet is its global reach. This is normally, and rightly, regarded as a great advantage. The downside, however, is that accusers can arise from anywhere and if that person is from a litigious society like the United States, then considerable difficulties can arise. This issue of liability to litigants in other countries is a fairly involved one and space does not permit me to do more than provide a bare summary. Not being resident in the litigant's country will often not give immunity: both UK law and our signatory status to several conventions governing international litigation may impose liability to a foreign litigant.

Some foreign laws present no real threat: tax and criminal laws are not directly applicable in the UK. Similarly, arbitrary foreign rules, such as failing to register with a health board, would not entitle that country to get extradition or allow it to recover a fine. Of course, it may pose difficulties if you were to travel there.

For a matter other than crime or tax, the picture becomes more complex. A number of requirements must be met for a foreign judgment to be enforceable: the court must be one that was entitled to make that judgment; the judgment must be final (i.e. not a temporary injunction); and it must be for a fixed sum of money.

Defences to the enforcement of such a judgment would be: that it was obtained in a breach of natural justice because the accused was not allowed to defend himself or herself; that it was obtained through fraud; that it was contrary to UK public policy; that it conflicted with another judgment on the same issue; that the court had no right to hear the case; that it conflicted with an agreement on where any disputes would be tried; that it would result in multiple damage awards for the same complaint; and finally that fresh evidence has been discovered.

The UK is a party to the Brussels and Lugano conventions. Under these it is obliged automatically to enforce judgments from other convention countries; however, limitations on the enforcement of judgments exist which are fairly similar to the usual English rules.

Depending on the practicalities of the case, it may be possible to have the venue moved to a UK court. This is obviously highly desirable, but it is important to get this question settled quickly rather than waiting, since once a court abroad has begun hearing the case it is much less likely that either the UK or foreign courts will accede to a request to have the case transferred to the UK.

Intellectual property

Varieties of intellectual property

In law, 'intellectual property' is an umbrella term that covers rights relating to the result of intellectual activity as well as non-physical property rights arising from doing trade. An example in the latter category would be the growing importance of, and conflicts surrounding, 'domain' names (the web addresses of organisations, such as *www.rcpsych.ac.uk*). Rights falling under the former category include patents and copyrights.

Copyright is a partial monopoly given for a period of time by the state to a person who, in the vocabulary of law, reduces an original idea to some form of fixed expression, that is, turns an idea into some permanent form. Thus an original novel, academic paper or computer program would, at the moment of writing, give the author the right to prevent others copying a substantial part of it for a period of 70 years from the death of the author. An impromptu talk would not be protected by copyright since it would never have been fixed in writing, nor would the mere idea for a book, since it would not have been written down.

In its everyday meaning 'originality' implies a quality judgement: novelty, imagination and great insight are called original. This approach is seen in the copyright laws of Germany and various countries that regard copyright as a reward for creativity and skill. However, in common law countries (mainly the UK, the US, Canada, Australia and Ireland) the approach is pragmatic and a very low level of creative originality is needed. For example, something as banal as a railway timetable is original enough to get copyright protection, even where it is generated automatically by a computer.

Infringement of copyright

Copyright gives a right to the owner of a copyright work to prevent reproductions or performances of the work. Ownership of the physical work is not the same as ownership of the copyright of the work embedded within it: being the owner of a CD means ownership just of the physical disk, not the rights in the music or software on it. However, copyright is not a monopoly right: two photographers can produce photographs of Big Ben that are indistinguishable but neither can prevent the other from selling his or her own version. By contrast a patent would allow only the person with the patent to exploit it commercially.

A law that prevented all copying would prevent many commonplace and important activities such as journalism, teaching and literary criticism, so copyright law incorporates common-sense provisions that allow the taking of non-substantial parts of a work. For example, quoting a sentence or two from someone else's paper at a conference would not be an infringement of copyright. There is, however, no fixed guide as to what is a fair amount to take when using someone else's work; sometimes taking large chunks of someone else's not very creative work is fine, but in other cases taking even of a paragraph from someone else's brilliant piece of research work would be infringing. What may be permissible is summarising someone else's work using sufficient of one's own words. This so-called 'fair dealing' – taking small parts of someone else's work – is both a measure of common sense and recognition that copying is, in truth, a source of inspiration in society. Many of the best and most popular works derive in part or in inspiration from copying the works of others; where would Disney be without the Brothers Grimm? Correct attribution, even in cases covered by 'fair dealing', is a legal necessity.

Liability for the copyright infringement of others

The law will sometimes impose liability on someone other than the primary infringer. This is currently being seen in the high-profile litigation against online music file-sharers in America. Usually the allegations are of 'vicarious' and 'contributory' infringement. In the UK this is called 'authorising infringement'. Collectively these are known as 'secondary infringement'. Typically in secondary infringement there is commercial dealing with a work where the copies in question are known or reasonably believed to be infringing copyright (e.g. selling pirated copies of a Madonna CD at a car boot sale).

The danger to employers or anyone responsible for another person's use of a computer is that, if that person engages in copyright infringement, for example by use of a file-sharing program, they may be liable. Indeed, it may even be the case that *criminal* liability arises.

Finally, the courts may refuse to enforce copyright in certain instances where there is criminality, immorality or an important issue of public policy; for example, if a criminal detailed exploits in a diary, then the courts would not allow him to use copyright law to prevent his public exposure.

Copyright law in the use of IT

The biggest legal risk in IT by far centres on software licensing. Software licences are necessary because running software entails making a transient copy of the program in the computer's memory: the copy of all or part of the program is read from a hard drive into the computer's memory. Without an end-user licence agreement (EULA) even this form of copying would be a breach of copyright law in most jurisdictions but not in the UK.

While most home users probably do not read the EULA and frequently use software without an appropriate licence, this is not the case in the world of business, where a trade association, the Business Software Alliance (BSA), aggressively enforces the copyrights of its members. One effective tool in the arsenal of the BSA is the use of informers, usually disgruntled ex-employees. In these cases fault does not always lie with the employer: it takes a great deal of administrative rigour and discipline to maintain an up-to-date and accurate inventory of licences. Furthermore, it is often the case that licences are thrown away or lost when office computers are changed. Even in an audit there is the practical difficulty of demonstrating that the software was lawfully obtained rather than being copied, or obtained at a car boot sale. There are software products that will automate the process of licence auditing to a degree but there is the need for formal and effectuated procedures to minimise this risk.

Another substantial risk is intentional or unintentional file sharing. A recent survey indicated that 33% of surveyed machines that were directly or indirectly connected to the internet were infected with viruses, Trojan horses or other malicious software, which are often used for such nefarious objectives as sending spam and transmitting pornography. Such machines typically display the outward appearance of normality but the risk exists that one day the police or some copyright protection agency will descend out of the blue because of these unseen activities.

Clearly then, there is the necessity for appropriate procedures relating to the installation of computer software. Users may be irritated by being unable to download a cool screensaver or a free game, but in a hostile world, where such things may contain viruses, a sensible policy that many IT systems administrators use is to lock down machines to pre-approved and verified packages. Additionally, many people keep the licences of all software they purchase, however old, in case they need to produce them.

A final option that may be worth considering is the use of 'open source' software. This is something of a new phenomenon in the software world and revolves around the apparently inverted principle of actively disclosing the 'crown jewels' of software: the source code. This enables collaborative development of software among an ad hoc network of individuals on the internet. The result is software that is often as good or indeed sometimes better than the commercial equivalent.

We have mentioned open-source alternatives such as the operating system and OpenOffice package at various places in this book. Many regard these products as at least equal to their commercial alternatives and often better, particularly in terms of stability and security. In addition, the software is usually available free or at a nominal price and there are no onerous and intrusive licensing requirements. This has not escaped the notice of cash-strapped governments around the world, including that of the UK.

Defamation

Defamation is the unjustified impugning of another's reputation, which causes that person damage. One of the perils of our interconnected world is the fact that publication can take place more easily than is generally imagined. An email intended for a colleague may be circulated to the wrong people. In catastrophic cases it may be even be circulated worldwide, as the author of the infamous 'Claire Squires' email found out. In his case an unhappy girlfriend and furious employer were the only consequences, but for a psychiatrist it could result in a professional disciplinary hearing or even expensive litigation. A casual aside to a colleague in a hospital corridor is one thing but when broadcast to the world it may become defamatory.

Lawyers alone love defamation cases. For example, after an online defamation Demon Internet had to pay £250 000 to a Mr Laurence Godfrey, of which only £15 000 was damages; the rest went in legal costs. Take an insider's advice: avoid defamation, unless you feel a moral obligation to put your lawyers children through private school!

The public policy aspects of defamation are significant owing to its limiting effect on free speech and its interplay with the subjective nature of reputation. Certain issues of public safety and public interest could be affected by defamation law. It is therefore an area of some controversy.

Defamation is not an action available to government bodies, local or national. Individual politicians, however, may sue if maligned.

Equally, if one has no reputation, then one cannot sue to defend it: this is the position of those with non-trivial criminal convictions. The same would be probably be true of a doctor convicted by a disciplinary panel.

Dissecting defamation

Defamation has two subgenres: slander and libel. Slander is where a defamatory statement is made in impermanent form, for example a spoken remark. Libel is a defamatory statement that is recorded in permanent form, such as writing. It is an approximate, and only approximate, rule of thumb that what is written is libellous and what is heard is slanderous.

A successful suit for libel does not require proof that the libelled person has been financially harmed by the libel. In the case of slander, however, such a financial loss must be demonstrated.

Libel is the most likely form of defamation on the internet, since it is still largely a textual medium, much of which is archived in the databases of internet search engines such as Google.

In contrast, ephemeral Internet media such as chat or instant messaging would seem to lend themselves more to claims of slander.

Defamation is a statement that has one of three effects: it lowers someone in the eyes of right-thinking people generally, or it subjects them to ridicule, hatred or contempt, or it causes them to be shunned or avoided.

Truth or falsehood has no relevance to whether a statement is defamatory or not. If you say of a colleague that he or she is inept, then the statement is defamatory and can be sued on. If it is false, the colleague is unjustly defamed and his or her reputation is wrongly damaged; if it is true, the colleague is defamed, albeit correctly, and everyone is warned of his or her ineptitude. In the case of the unjust accusation there is no defence, since the statement is false, while where the statement is true the defence of justification is available. From this definition it should also be clear that merely insulting someone is not defamatory so long as the insult contains nothing amounting to a factual accusation.

What if you want to wound but fear to strike? Is it safe to drop hints? Words can have several meanings, some good, some bad and some with a meaning known only to insiders. If instead of describing a colleague as inept you had chosen to say he or she was ‘trusting’, might that not be rather a good thing in a doctor? It might not be if, for example, the doctor in question was tasked with performing risk assessments in a forensic context. If defamatory words bear an alternative meaning or a meaning understood by only a few, then a judge will have to decide whether the words were capable of having that defamatory meaning. If the judge thinks they can, then a jury will be allowed to decide whether they actually were defamatory.

Viewers of the television series *Have I Got News For You* will be familiar with panellists uttering defamatory-sounding remarks prefaced with ‘it is alleged that’. There is a widespread belief that this liturgy is garlic to repel the vampyric defamation lawyer. Alas, repeating defamation as a report of an allegation amounts to a republication of it and is a fresh cause of action.

Different audiences can also have different values. To say of someone that he or she was a papist might not boil the blood now but several centuries ago in Britain it might have resulted in imprisonment and torture. These values fade over time and eventually they lose their defamatory barb.

Male homosexuality is now lawful, but since many people still regard this as aberrant behaviour Tom Cruise was able to sue, successfully, for these allegations, protesting all the way to the bank that there was, none the less, nothing wrong with being gay.

Just as truth is a defence to defamation so is fair comment. This is perhaps as well, since in the previous paragraph I wrote of Tom Cruise that he 'was able to sue, successfully, for these allegations, protesting all the way to the bank that there was, none the less, nothing wrong with being gay'.

We've discussed the danger of defamation as a limit on free speech. If what is said can be viewed as an opinion rather than a statement of fact, it should be permissible, so as to reduce the risk of damage to free speech. The exact dividing line between fact and opinion can be vague, but defamation law generally takes the view that if what is said is a conclusion or evaluation based on facts then it is opinion, but if it invites the reader to make a conclusion then it is a statement of fact.

Clearly, carelessness in fact-gathering is also a danger; fair comment on inaccurate facts would be an invitation, indeed a compulsion, to the media to be inaccurate and careless in order to safeguard itself. The defence requires that if the comment is shaky at least its foundations need to be secure. Since the role of this defence is primarily that of a safety valve for democratic debate, it is necessary for the comment to be about things either in the public interest or of interest to the public. Were it otherwise many a tabloid paper's Sunday edition would be rather thin. Thus, suggesting hypocrisy by a famous film star is an evaluative comment based on accurate fact and so I, and the publishers of this book, are safe.

There is also the obvious need that the statement should to refer to the person defamed. In defamation law the test of whom the statement refers to is an objective one, in which intent plays no part. This is illustrated by the case of *Hulton* v. *Jones*, in which the plaintiff had the same name as someone accused of adultery. Despite the similar names, very little else was comparable between the fictional and real Jones, but it was decided that the test was whether the reader would believe they were the same person and in the case the answer was yes. Newspapers address this by danger by being more specific in identifying whom it is they are talking about, so now, for example, rather than talking of Mr Jones, they talk of Mr Artemis Jones, a lawyer of Acacia Avenue.

The final requirement of defamation is that the allegation is published to someone else. Some people do not count and you can publish to them without fear; these include the person defamed, the partner of the defamer and also someone who cannot understand what is said (perhaps because they speak only another language).

It may also be that one did not intend to publish the statement but unforeseen events caused it to be published. The question to be asked is whether those events were foreseeable in the normal course of events.

It should be noted in passing that every republication is a fresh defamation, so everyone from the author to the publisher to the person handing it out on the street is potentially liable. This fairly strict position should be contrasted with the situation in other countries, such as the United States, where there is liability only if they knew of the content. In the UK there is a defence of innocent dissemination that is similar in effect, except that it is a defence to be proven, rather than a burden the accuser must overcome.

In even more liberal jurisdictions secondary publishers are liable only if they change the communication. As we shall see later, this has significance for free speech on the English portion of the internet and it has caused problems for English publishers.

Defeating a defamation action

However risky defamation may be, there are some who are immune. Speakers in Parliament have absolute immunity from defamation actions, as a result of the 1688 Bill of Rights. Absolute privilege also applies in court cases so long as what is said is connected with the case and the hearing is of a judicial rather than administrative character. Forensic evidence given by a psychiatrist in court would have such protection. However, such evidence given by a psychiatrist in, say, an adoption case or a housing benefit case might not be, since those would be hearings of an administrative rather than judicial character. Even in administrative cases it might be possible to persuade a court to grant an immunity if the absence of protection would seriously hamper an important public function.

A slightly weaker form of the 'absolute privilege' defence exists called 'qualified privilege'. The characteristic difference here is that it applies generally to the reporting of parliamentary and court proceedings, provided that the reporting is fair, accurate and not malicious. Here 'malicious' has a specific legal meaning: not believing or caring whether what was said was true; being reckless about its truth or falsity; acting with a motive other than the doing one's duty or protecting one's own interests or the interests of the person the remark is made to.

This class of defence is quite important in practice. For example, when giving references for colleagues or co-workers there is clearly a risk of making a defamatory statement by mistake. If that remark is not true, the main plank of one's defence would be to say that the prospective employer needs to know that there are substantial accusations of dishonesty or incompetence about that person, and so long as there is no malice this defence may work. Similarly, reporting a patient's suspected criminal conduct to the police would probably be defensible, again, so long as the accusation was not malicious.

Remedies for defamation

Damages

Traditionally, defamation cases led, in some instances, to the payment of enormous sums in damages. The sums involved sometimes dwarfed those paid for causing serious physical injury and disability. The fact that the amount of damages, or 'quantum', was usually decided in defamation cases by the jury rather than the judge might have contributed to the large awards. This has recently changed and if an award is either excessive or inadequate the judge can substitute what he or she feels is a proper sum.

Injunctions

An injunction is an effective means to prevent a wrong or limit damage. Injunctions tend not to be granted where money would be a better remedy, but a reputation when lost is usually lost for good. Since money may not be an adequate compensation for this damage an injunction will often be obtainable. The remedy is often particularly effective since to disobey it would be a contempt of court, which may result in imprisonment and fines. An additional incentive with injunctions is that, in practice, after being granted they often tend to end the matter in dispute.

Defamation meets the internet

Defamation committed online is not conceptually different from that committed elsewhere and it is now well established by case law that electronic defamation is equivalent to any other form.

Chat forums

The web has allowed ordinary people to bypass publishers, media barons and government censors and get their message out to the world. While this has been an empowering and democratic revolution, like all revolutions it has some downsides, of which defamation is one.

Web forums and email consistently give rise to accusations of defamation and it is a threat that is even more potent to individuals who may lack the legal advice available to conventional publishers, who have professional experience and a greater ability to meet the costs of that advice.

Some types of forum are easier to control than others; the so-called blog (a contraction of 'web' and 'log') is usually published by one person, who may or may not allow others to comment on entries. This is a moderated type of forum since the blog owner makes the decision to publish remarks or permit the publication of comments.

Other forums, such as web-based chat rooms and Usenet discussion groups, are far less regulated. The latter pre-date the web and use different technical mechanisms, but in essence comprise a series of topic-based conversation groups arranged in a hierarchical structure. Examples include *alt.psychology, alt.psychology.jung, alt.psychology.psychoanalysis*.

These discussion groups are not located on any one computer or under the control of any one institution, hence it is virtually impossible to withdraw a published message. It was in one such forum that the best-known British internet defamation case arose. A physics lecturer by the name of Godfrey participated in discussions within the *forum alt.soc.thai*. A dispute appears to have arisen with other forum participants and an unknown individual in America posted a defamatory remark, which began to propagate to various different Usenet servers around the world.

In the UK, Demon Internet was one of the internet service providers that carried the group and it refused to remove the offending message when Godfrey complained to it, as the company claimed that it, like the telephone company, was merely a conduit for messages. It was held, however, that, by refusing to remove the message when informed, it had republished it to its users. Demon had to pay some £250 000 to Godfrey in costs and damages.

A couple of observations can be drawn from this case. First, if participating in professional forums, then it is clear that an off-the-cuff remark can be misinterpreted and that it may be tremendously difficult or impossible to retract it. It is clear that a person who is defamed and who acts quickly in complaining to an internet service provider may reduce the damage suffered and decrease the circulation of the message. Second, those in charge of such a forum need an effective mechanism for reacting quickly and effectively to abuse.

Email

An email may be misdirected by a single mouse click but the consequences may spiral rapidly out of control. Emails about colleagues or patients intended only for internal circulation may reach the inbox of the person concerned.

The above-mentioned 'Claire Squires' email from, of all places, a law firm, detailed the sexual behaviour of named individuals and caused controversy for all involved, including the employer. In part this is an issue of data protection, a matter we discussed earlier in this chapter, but the contents may also be defamatory. For example, if a diagnosis falls into the wrong hands, civil liability will rest on whether there was a breach of data protection rules, or there was negligence or defamation. In respect of the latter cause of action it is probable that there is a defence of either justification or, at worst, qualified privilege since the person to whom the email is directed is likely to have a proper interest in the patient, perhaps as a fellow healthcare professional.

If it is not possible for a plaintiff to sue for defamation then an action in negligence may still be feasible. The argument would be that a duty of care was breached by inadvertence in the use of email and that damage was suffered as a result. Public key encryption, as described by Mike Madden in Chapter 13, would prevent emails being read by people other than the intended recipient. While many email encryption systems are difficult to use and the supporting infrastructure is not well developed, it is likely that encryption will eventually play an important role in confidential medical communications; indeed, it may become a requirement if liability is to be avoided.

Crime and punishment

Pornography is perhaps the highest-profile computer crime, followed closely by hacking. Scarcely a week goes by without tabloid headlines about a paedophile being caught with a hard disk full of compromising images. In addition, computers are frequently used as tools to aid other offences, such as harassment, fraud and acts of racial hatred. In the domain of psychiatry the problems that are most likely to arise relate to patients, although the acts of staff also need to be considered.

The basis of criminal liability

Most psychiatrists will know, from their medico-legal work, that a criminal conviction requires that the accused commits the guilty act in question (the *actus reus*) and also has the intent to do so (the *mens rea*). There are a few, relatively minor, offences where this is not the case (strict liability).

Professional risk

Aiding and abetting

Imagine the situation where a forensic in-patient is given unsupervised access to the internet and uses it to 'groom' a child or download child pornography. Might the responsible doctor also be prosecuted for criminal negligence, or for aiding and abetting?

In English law a person who, in the language of the Accessories and Abettors Act 1861, 'aids, abets, counsels, and procures' the commission of an indictable act is liable as though he or she were the person doing the act. In law this is examined in two ways: to aid and abet one needs to be present at the scene of the act and offer at least minimal encouragement, while to 'counsel and procure' one need not be present but previous encouragement should have been offered. In both cases the encouragement needs to have happened before the main criminal act occurred and not after it. In a scenario where encouragement is needed it is rather difficult to see how liability could realistically be imposed on a doctor and the main risk is probably to one who is tardy in taking corrective action.

In most situations there is no legal obligation (although there may be a moral one) to come to the assistance of another person in jeopardy. However, the law *will* impose a duty to intervene in some cases, such as those where there is a domestic or professional obligation of care. For example, a parent is obliged to care for a child and a doctor is not entitled to stand aside while a patient under his or her care is either neglected by or abuses others; where such an obligation of responsibility arises the position is different and one can be an accessory by mere inaction.

Criminal negligence

Another source of risk is the issue of negligence. Civil liability for negligence is discussed above but where the inadvertence is gross it may justify criminal charges. This is a charge that has been laid against doctors at various times, although more typically in the setting of non-psychiatric cases. In the case of *R* v. *Adamako* a locum anaesthetist failed to resuscitate a patient. He was prosecuted and convicted; he then appealed to the House of Lords. They confirmed that the elements of the offence were:

- the existence of a duty of care
- a breach of that duty, causing death
- gross negligence, which the jury considered justified a criminal conviction.

It is for the jury to make a finding of gross negligence if the evidence shows that the defendant:

- was indifferent to an obvious risk of injury
- had foresight of the risk but determined nevertheless to run it
- appreciated the risk and intended to avoid it but displayed a high degree of negligence in the attempted avoidance
- displayed inattention to a serious risk, or otherwise failed to avert it, that went beyond 'mere inadvertence' in respect of an obvious and important matter which the defendant's duty demanded he or she should address.

How would this be likely to affect a psychiatrist in the context of technology? The risk is certainly a real one, given the example above. In the first instance there will clearly be a need for risk assessment and this will primarily be the duty of the relevant hospital trust or management.

It would, however, be dangerous for a psychiatrist to do nothing because of a lack of management motivation or his or her own technical inability. The risk is that a court would not view this hesitance as acceptable and it might say that the doctor should have undertaken, at the very least, minimal precautions or have obtained technical help to do so. In any event, the sort of procedures that would need to be examined would address issues relating to paedophile activity or stalking and sexual or racial harassment, in addition to the classic issues of IT security (those relating to viruses and passwords, for example). In truth, however, the risks in most cases are minimal because, as discussed above, to convict there is the requirement for a guilty mind. Even serious negligence or poor judgement is unlikely to be sufficient.

Obscenity

Obscenity is perhaps the highest-profile offence committed with computers. Under the Obscene Publications Act 1959 the possession or distribution for profit of obscene materials is an offence and the test of obscenity is whether the material is likely to deprave or corrupt. This does require an intent to profit, which is not usually present in a clinical setting.

Other offences under the Protection of Children Acts 1976 and 1978 may have more relevance, for example those relating to the making, possessing or distributing of indecent images. Typically, prosecutions have related to indecent images of children, although animal rights posters or anything else that 'offends against the modesty of the average man' may be held to be obscene. Charges that are laid against accused persons usually derive from section 160 of the Criminal Justice Act 1988 and are framed in terms of 'making' images in the sense of a photographic modelling session.

Recent cases relating to child and adult pornography have given a rather strained and literal definition to the word, whereby recording on to a computer hard drive amounts to 'making' an image. In a literal sense this is true but this 'making' is usually an automatic one, removed from any deliberate action of the user; for example, web browsers automatically store website images in a cache for the sake of efficiency – the user never does this knowingly and most are not even aware it happens.

The offence of indecency is measured against standards of propriety at the lower end of the scale; but how far such an image has to sink below these low standards is unclear and is dependent on the particular facts. In the words of one judge: 'I cannot define obscenity but I know it when I see it'.

The ability of computers to create stunningly realistic simulations can be seen every day in films such as *Lord of the Rings*. Almost inevitably, this capability has been perverted to produce obscene materials such as realistic paedophilic images. In some countries these are lawful on the basis that no real children were involved, or that no real abuse took place; in other jurisdictions the argument that they are none the less criminally unacceptable and may encourage or reinforce aberrant behaviour has prevailed. The UK falls into the latter category and amended legislation on the protection of children outlaws synthetic obscenity, on pain of distinctly non-synthetic penalties.

Section 160(2)(a) of the Criminal Justice Act 1988 provides that 'Where a person is charged with an offence under ss(1) above, it shall be a defence for him to prove – (a) that he had a legitimate reason for having the photograph or pseudo-photograph in his possession'. So a police officer might lawfully possess such images and a psychologist or psychiatrist possessing such images for clinical reasons would also have a defence.

'Where did that come from?'

One of the difficulties of computers is that most people do not have an intimate understanding of their inner workings; when coupled with the false veneer of internet anonymity it has led to the downfall of many a pornographer. Forensic computer specialists can often recover files believed by the user to be deleted but which the computer has, in reality, merely marked as invisible pending deletion. Similarly, most web browsers will 'cache' (store) downloaded graphics in a dark corner of the computer so that they need not be downloaded a second time if that site is revisited. For the fan of pornography this poses a danger, since these caches are hard to find for those not in the know – but that category rarely includes police forensic specialists. However, since all images are cached without user intervention it may well be that someone misdirected to a website, perhaps by a spam email or a virus, may inadvertently download and 'make' such material, and risk criminal conviction.

A more insidious threat arises from so-called Trojan programs, which are a form of malicious software that allows a distant person to use a computer without the knowledge of the owner. Trojans have been used recently to send untraceable spam email or as launch pads for attacks on other systems. The purpose of this is to disguise the origin of the true attacker, since any analysis of the network traffic will show the infected computer as the originator of the attack and not the address of the true perpetrator.

To date there is no evidence that Trojans are routinely used to disseminate child pornography but Trojans have occasionally downloaded it; in July and August 2003 in separate court cases two men were acquitted of criminal charges when compelling forensic evidence supported their assertions that Trojans had downloaded the images.

Trojan infections are rapidly increasing and pose perhaps the greatest current threat that needs to be addressed.

Responding to the threat

In a clinical context, these risks arise from inadequate policies and inadequate supervision. These can be largely resolved with appropriate advice from IT support groups, together with legal advice on monitoring policy from a hospital trust's legal department. It may be felt that patients and staff need access to PCs, but if so then some minimal methods of security can be implemented that should involve monitoring of internet usage such as web surfing and email. This can be accomplished by technical means using software that logs access to the internet.

Antivirus software, when regularly updated, should be able to deal with the great majority of Trojans and worms. Only authorised users with individual passwords should have access to machines.

Such policies and technical measures, however, need to be implemented in a manner that is sensitive to the privacy of users, particularly in the context of the Human Rights Act.

Dealing with criminal acts

Surprisingly there is no general duty to report the commission of an offence, or the suspicion of one, to the police. Exceptions exist in relation to terrorism and money laundering, but a clinician discovering crime, say as a result of counselling, need not report it to the police if he or she does not wish to. Indeed, there may be good reason not to do so if it would compound the harm to the patient or others, or damage a professional relationship. For example, vulnerable individuals often complain that being a witness in a criminal prosecution is a distressing experience despite attempts by the police to be sensitive. If this were felt to risk adverse health consequences to a patient, then that would seem to be an acceptable reason for not making a complaint .

Conversely, there is nothing to prevent a clinician reporting an offence or suspected offence regardless of the patient's wishes. If a patient reports an act of abuse, then that is sensitive and confidential information that would ordinarily attract an obligation of confidentiality. However, if the matter is criminal, then there is a countervailing public policy imperative and it is unlikely that reporting it to the police would be unlawful. It is hard to imagine that a patient who confessed to a doctor that he was a rapist would have any basis for a successful legal action against the clinician. Furthermore, if the police have a firm basis for a suspicion it may be possible for them to persuade a court to issue an injunction instructing the holder of information to disclose it; however, principles of medical confidentiality would usually make this a fairly substantial burden for them to overcome.

Conclusion

It is my hope that this chapter has helped to clarify the legal risks associated with the increasing use of IT in mental health. It is not my intention, however, to discourage innovation in this area as IT, properly deployed, has great potential to improve service delivery and patient care.

CHAPTER 13

Keeping your computers secure

Michael G. Madden

As a psychiatrist, you doubtless have a filing cabinet in your office that contains highly confidential information, so you keep it locked, you keep the office locked in the security-patrolled office building and you are very careful about whom you give access to the keys.

But what about the computer in your office? Unfortunately, the physical building security provides only one, very small part of the overall security infrastructure required. This chapter will help you to understand the potential security vulnerabilities and how to overcome them. The topics discussed reflect the different levels of responsibility for computers you have in the multiple roles you may play: as an employee of a hospital or clinic; as a manager of a hospital unit; as an employer within your private practice; and as a home user.

This chapter addresses the issue of data security; it will help you to identify potential vulnerabilities to data loss (either malicious or accidental) and data theft, and provide you with simple strategies for guarding against them.

What data are the most important to protect? Many of the files on your computer will be less important from a security perspective than others. Here's a simple exercise. Look at a list of files on your computer, and for each one ask yourself whether it would be a big problem if either it vanished or someone else (e.g. colleagues, journalists, patients, ex-patients) read it. For some files, one of these will matter much more than the other.

All the topics discussed here will deserve attention if you wish to make your computer relatively secure. A checklist is provided at the end.

Backups

Most of this chapter is concerned with guarding your computer against [illegible] theft. However, protecting against data loss is also important. Disks or [illegible] components can fail; laptops get stolen or lost; some viruses delete [illegible] repairs and software upgrades can go wrong; and users sometimes overwrite or delete files accidentally.

If you work in a hospital or clinic where you are an employee, then you should be able simply to use that organisation's backup procedures for your office computer. You will need to inform yourself of these procedures and apply them. You may, for example, have to install software on your computer, leave the computer on at night, and/or store files to be backed up in a specific folder. Check with the organisation's system administrator.

However, you still will have to take responsibility for backing up your laptop, your home PC and the PC in your private practice, if you have one. In that case, there are three important issues to consider:

- What should you back up?
- How will you back it up?
- How do you protect the backups?

What should you back up?

You need to back up any files that would cause you problems if they were lost. For most of us, this means documents that we have written and received, and our email. You don't need to back up local copies of journal papers that you have downloaded, as you could retrieve them from the original source if they were lost. Nor do you need to back up your operating system files or program files, as you should be able to reinstall them. For many users only 10–20% of disk space may be taken up with files that need backing up, although it may be more convenient to back up everything.

Of course, every time you alter a file, you need to back up the changed version. It can be disheartening to realise, when you've lost a document that you've worked on solidly for a week, that the newest backup is 5 days old.

How will you back it up?

There are two approaches to making backups: manually or using backup software. The manual approach is simply to copy important files to a storage device such as a tape drive, a CD or DVD or a server on the network. National Health Service staff are usually encouraged to save important files to a network drive in the first place and while this offers automatic backup assurance – information technology (IT) support staff will usually back up network drives – it can mean that files are hard to access if the network is having problems.

This manual approach is OK for making ad hoc backups of important documents, but if you want to put in place a comprehensive backup procedure for your computer, it is easier and more reliable to use backup software.

The first point to decide is what storage device to use for backups. The key issue here is storage capacity. The classic backup devices are DAT tape drives and Zip drives, but CD writers are popular now as they have quite high capacity (650 MB) and rewritable disks (CD-RW) are cheap. DVD disks are slightly more expensive, but have capacities of over 4500 MB. New PCs come with one or the other. Another option becoming popular is the USB drive (see Chapter 9). These compact devices plug into a USB port on your computer and function as removable disk drives.

The features you should look for in a backup program include:

- easy-to-use graphical user interfaces for backups and restores
- support for incremental and multi-level backups
- automatic scheduling of backups, so you don't have to remember to run backups and so they can be run overnight
- facilities for backing up system settings, such as program configurations and mail settings.

The idea of incremental backups is that you back up your whole system the first time, but the next time you back up only those files that have changed since the last backup. However, you have to alternate between incremental and full backups: if you just keep making repeated incremental backups, then when you need to restore files you will have to search through all your old backup disks – one of which might be missing or overwritten.

Multi-level backups are better: you occasionally (maybe once per year) perform a level-0 backup of the whole hard drive; monthly, you perform a level-1 backup of everything that has changed since the last level-0 backup; and daily, you perform a level-2 backup of everything that has changed since the last level-1 backup.

A different approach is taken by software that 'mirrors' or clones specified folders onto a separate storage drive, which could be a CD-RW, a USB drive or a second computer. The first time it is run, all files in specified folders are duplicated. Afterwards, the software checks for additions, deletions or changes, and duplicates these. This gives a good level of protection, particularly if you mirror files to a computer in a different room. Of course, both computers can operate as mirrors for each other, or you can use an old PC as the mirror for all others. It is important to configure the software to keep copies of old files, to guard against accidental deletions. Combining this with periodic full backups gives even greater security.

Windows XP includes a program called Windows Backup, which has all of the basic features listed above, apart from multi-level backups. Its biggest drawback is that it cannot write to CDs or DVDs. Several other inexpensive backup programs do support removable disks.

How do you protect the backups?

One of the reasons to make backups is so that you can get your data back in the unlikely event that your computer is stolen or damaged in a fire. Therefore, it is not a very good idea to leave the backup disk on top of your monitor when you're finished.

You'll also need to guard against theft. Physical PC security is discussed below. However, data thieves won't need to attack your computer if you've left a backup disk lying around with all the good stuff.

The accepted solution is to store your backups off-site. For example, you could keep your office computer backups at home. It's best to purchase a small fire-proof safe for keeping the backups in, and stash it in a different room. A more secure, but less convenient, alternative is to keep backups in a safety deposit box at a bank.

As a final safeguard, you should check whether your backup software supports password protection or backup encryption. If it does, use these features, as they will make life more difficult for a thief who steals your backup disks.

Online backup services

An interesting trend is the emergence of online backup service providers. These companies provide small offices and home users with a backup service analogous to the institutional backup procedures available in large organisations. Typically, you are provided with a program to install on your computer. Using this, you specify what files/folders you want to back up and what schedule you want to follow. At the times you have chosen, the backup program starts up and transfers your files across the internet to a server belonging to the backup company.

There are several advantages to online backup services. The most important one is, of course, that the day-to-day responsibility for organising and managing backups becomes somebody else's problem! Other benefits are:

- You don't have to invest a lump sum in backup software or storage devices.
- You will be able to restore files that you overwrote or deleted days or months ago.
- Dedicated backup companies can provide extremely high levels of security: backup servers in bunkers; duplicate copies in centres hundreds of miles apart; security guard patrols; and so on.
- Backups can even be restored from a different computer, which could be useful even if you have not lost files. For example, when travelling you could retrieve a copy of a file that's on your home PC from the backup server.

There are, though, a couple of drawbacks:

- *Cost*. Over time, the monthly subscription would exceed the lump-sum cost of hardware and software to do it yourself. Of course, you are getting a different service.
- *Bandwidth*. You definitely need an always-on broadband internet connection, because of the amount of data that you will have to upload to the

backup server. Even at that, home broadband services typically have much higher download speeds than upload speeds, but with an online backup service you'll be uploading all the data to back up. This could represent a significant additional cost.

A final note of caution: choose your backup service provider carefully. Be aware of the legal issues discussed in Chapter 12 and ensure that the provider you choose has the technical and legal guards in place to guarantee that nobody can access your data on its server.

Passwords

Passwords are ubiquitous. You need them to log on to each computer you use, to connect to your internet service, to access your mail, even to remember your preferences when you're shopping online. You can even password-protect individual documents, as we'll see later.

The use of 'good' or 'strong' passwords is the first step in protecting your data's confidentiality and integrity. However, to maintain your data's availability, you must be able to recall the password when you need it. Good passwords, therefore, are easy for you to remember but difficult for anybody else to guess, and are changed regularly.

How can my password be discovered?

There are many ways your password can be discovered. It can be guessed very easily if it's your pet's name, your date of birth or any other piece of publicly known information about you. It can also be guessed if it's a common word; 'fred' is popular, as the letters occur together on the keyboard – people staring at the keyboard looking for inspiration may think of it without even noticing this. Apparently, among male executives in particular, 'god' is a common choice (don't ask me why, you're the psychiatrist!).

There are many password-cracking programs that try thousands of passwords until they find one that works. These are generally based on dictionaries in one or multiple languages, along with lists of names of people and places. Some even enumerate all possible combinations of four or even more letters.

A cracker with physical access to your computer can look around: passwords are often written on notes stuck to the monitor or under the keyboard, or in a nearby diary or address book (most likely under 'P', lest the cracker's life be made too difficult!). This is the electronic equivalent of leaving your house key under the doormat.

Another popular storage place is on the computer itself, listed among reminders or email contacts. This is as bad or worse.

External computers such as your email server store a copy of your password so that it can verify when you enter your password that it is correct. Normally, such servers encrypt passwords, but not all are equally secure. Some web servers are particularly poorly designed and even store passwords as plain text. If such a server is attacked, and you have used the same password for that website as for your computer login, this could give the cracker access to much more interesting information. In general, you should not use the same password for different purposes. After all, it wouldn't be very secure to have a single key that worked for your office, your house, your new car and your gym locker!

Some types of Trojan (see below) include keystroke loggers so an external individual can discover everything you type.

Finally, some crackers don't bother stealing passwords; they just ask for them! By pretending to be a systems administrator or some other responsible person, they can often persuade innocent users to part with private information. This is discussed in more detail below.

Guidelines for good passwords

Consideration of how bad practice can be exploited to discover your passwords should help you remember the following pointers:

- Pick passwords that are longer than eight characters.
- Include a mixture of upper-case letters, lower-case letters, digits and punctuation.
- Don't base your password on easily discovered personal information.
- Don't use a single word from any language, although a phrase like 'cAts+2+thE+rEscUE' is fine.
- Use different passwords for different purposes: your home, work and other computer logins, your email access and access to various websites.
- Treat your passwords like your toothbrush: change them regularly and never share them with anybody!

If, like me, you're the kind of person who has to look up your own mobile phone number when somebody asks for it, your reaction to these guidelines will probably be: 'Fine, but there's no way I'm going to remember eight different, complicated, frequently changing passwords. I'll just stick to using "fred" for the lot of them, and hope for the best.' With that in mind, I've come up with a suggestion for making the process a whole lot simpler.

Picking hard passwords made easy

Every month or two, pick an interesting journal or newspaper article. Cut it out and paste it on the wall by your desk. Base your passwords on patterns of letters from this article: for example, your email password might be generated from the third letter of every third line. When you change the article you'll have to change the passwords to match, but you can keep the same pattern. Just make sure you never disclose the pattern to anybody. If you must take note of it, write it on paper and store it in a safe.

There are several benefits to this. First and most importantly, you will generate passwords that are long, seemingly random (unless the third letter of every third line happens to spell out your cat's name!), and include a mix of letters and punctuation. However, they will still be easy for you to verify, so that you can avoid the sinking feeling that comes from using complex passwords: 'Hang on, is it "Ay9Sfaf5693hhy" or "Ay9sfaf5963hhy"?' Second, the article date gives you an easy way to check how old the password is. Third, you can generate all of your passwords just by using different patterns in the same article. Fourthly, if you pick an article that's available online, for example, you should be able to check up on passwords even if you're out of the office. Finally, even if somebody suspects that your password is based on the article pinned on your wall, without knowing the pattern they will be highly unlikely to be able to guess it.

Incidentally, this rather cheeky strategy of hiding highly confidential information by putting it in plain view but buried in irrelevant 'noise' is an ancient technique called steganography, which has received renewed attention in recent years. Many counter-terrorism experts believe that terrorist organisations are actively using steganographic techniques to exchange hidden messages embedded in innocuous-looking websites.

Physical security

Rather than attack your computer across a network, some data thieves go directly to the source computer. If you have an office where patients or other people can pass by, you probably would not leave a particularly sensitive patient file on your desk if you stepped out for a couple of minutes. You have to be equally vigilant with your desktop PC, if it contains electronic versions of many of your sensitive files.

In addition to the measures discussed below, you also need to consider the physical security of removable storage, such as CD-RW disks, tapes and USB drives.

User logins and passwords

The first line of defence is to protect your computer as you protect your filing cabinet – lock the office when you leave it. Of course, there is also a lock on the filing cabinet itself, to prevent somebody who has legitimate or unauthorised access to an office key from browsing it. Therefore, the second line of defence is having a strong, frequently changed login password. In fact, a login password is essential, as it is your first line

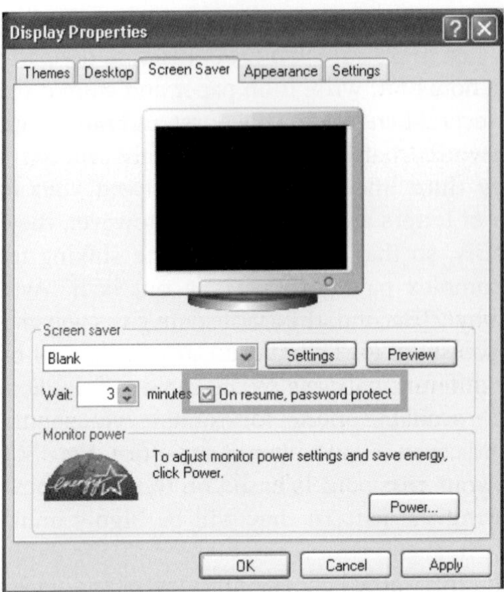

Fig. 13.1 Enabling the screen saver password.

of defence from crackers who attack your computer across a network. Unfortunately, some versions of Microsoft Windows do not require you to log in at all: anybody can just turn on your computer (or possibly connect to it across the network) and start using it. This is a bad idea; if your computer is like this, you should immediately set up a login account for yourself via the User Accounts setting on the Control Panel. To avoid anybody using your login account, you should log out when you finish using your computer.

As you will undoubtedly leave your computer unattended occasionally, you should enable your screensaver password. On Windows, for example, this is done using **Start → Control Panel → Display Properties**. Figure 13.1 shows this setting as it appears in Windows XP. For maximum effectiveness, you should set your screensaver so that it kicks in after a short duration.

BIOS passwords

By their nature, laptops are naturally more prone to theft than desktop PCs. Kensington locks are useful for chaining your laptop or data projector to the desk if you have to leave it unattended.

Your laptop's BIOS password provides additional security (the basic input/output system or BIOS is, if you like, the autonomic nervous system of your computer). This is a password that must be entered when you power up the computer. If it's wrong, the laptop will shut itself down. The procedure for setting a BIOS password depends on the computer model;

you should consult your computer manual or search for 'brand name bios password' on the web. Unfortunately, if you do a search like that, you'll be depressed to discover that for every web page with helpful advice on how to set your BIOS password, there are 20 with equally helpful device on how circumvent the BIOS password if you have 'forgotten' it. So, as throughout this chapter, multiple layers of security must be used.

Who has physical access to your computer?

To conclude this section, it may be worthwhile to consider who may be able physically to access to your computer. In your office block, maintenance and security personnel will have keys to your office, and it is possible that another person could get access to them. A zealous attacker might even remove your computer's hard drive and connect it to a different computer, to circumvent passwords. Consider file encryption, discussed below, to help frustrate such attacks.

In another category are people to whom you willingly give your computer, such as repair people. Remember that they will have a high level of technical knowledge! Apparently, the favourite pastime of some is to rummage through customers' file systems. As well as looking at the files you know about, they may look in obscure places, such as the cache of web sites that you've visited recently. They may also run 'undelete' utilities to recover files that you thought you had got rid of. In one case, a British performer was charged with possession of child pornography after he had left his computer in a shop for upgrading, and technicians found incriminating images in his web cache.

If you have sensitive patient information in unencrypted form on your malfunctioning computer, you might be advised to supervise the computer technicians who repair it, or assign somebody trustworthy to do so for you.

Communications security

It is of course essential for practising psychiatrists to be able to communicate securely with each other. The linchpin of modern communications is email. When exchanging email messages with a colleague, you may well want to do one or both of the following:

1 digitally sign messages and their attachments, providing a guarantee that the message did indeed come from you and was not tampered with in transit;
2 encrypt messages and their attachments, to ensure that nobody can view the message during transit.

The techniques for digital signatures and encryption that I'll describe in this section are based on a standard called S/MIME. This is the most widely used email security standard, and is supported by the popular email applications, including Microsoft Outlook, Microsoft Outlook Express, Netscape Mail, Mozilla Thunderbird, Pine and Eudora (with an appropriate 'plug-in'). Of the email applications I have tested, my opinion is that Netscape 7.1 Mail and the closely related Thunderbird (both of which are free) provide the best support for these features: they attach obvious icons to digitally signed and secure messages, and clearly explain the security aspects of messages. Basic use of the Thunderbird email client is covered in Chapter 11.

Encryption and digital signatures

The main motivation behind encryption of email messages is the realisation that when I send a message to you, it passes through a sequence of mail servers, each of which stores and forwards it to the next. A cracker who has access to any server along the route could intercept, read and even tamper with the message.

This also provides some of the motivation behind digital signatures, since they prevent tampering. However, the main motivation for digital signatures is that the 'from' field in an email message is extremely easy to fake: when you create an email account, your mail program will ask you to enter your email address as it will appear when messages are sent to other people, and there's nothing to keep you from entering *prime-minister@number-10.gov.uk* or *beckham@real.es*.

Digital signatures have been given recognition under law in most countries, so that a digital signature is regarded as legal proof that a message is authentic (i.e. came from whom it claims to come from), has not been tampered with, and cannot be repudiated (the sender cannot plausibly deny sending it).

Both security measures – encryption and digital signatures – are based on a technology called public key cryptography, briefly described below. From a practical point of view, all you need to do is get a digital certificate. Then you can go ahead with attaching digital signatures to messages and encrypting them too.

Public key cryptography

The whole purpose of cryptography is to be able to encrypt information (files, email messages, etc.) so that only nominated people can decrypt it. Before the invention of public key cryptography, you would scramble a file with a secret password (your key) and transmit the file to the recipient, who would unscramble it using the same password. Of course, you would first have to transmit your secret password to the recipient, which was the great weakness of such approaches.

Public key cryptography does not have this weakness. Instead, thanks to a bit of mathematical magic, you use two passwords (keys) that are different but complementary: if a message is scrambled with either one of the keys, it can be unscrambled only using the other key. Then, one of the keys is designated as your private key (which you must not disclose to anybody) and the other one as your public key (which you tell the whole world about).

Thus, if somebody wants to send you a message for your eyes only, they use your public key to encrypt the message, knowing that only you have the other key required to decrypt it.

Conversely, to digitally sign a message, you send it twice: once in plain text and once encrypted with your private key. Then, anybody can verify that it came from you and has not been tampered with, just by decrypting the encrypted version using your public key and verifying that this matches the plain-text version.

In practice, of course, all the encryption, decryption and verification is handled automatically by your email application once you own a pair of keys.

Certification authorities and getting a digital certificate

Public and private keys are issued by a certification authority (CA), which creates a digital certificate (or digital ID) for you that itself is digitally signed by the CA and contains information such as:

- your name and email address
- your public key
- the expiry date of the certificate
- details about the CA.

Two of the best-known CAs internationally are VeriSign and Thawte. These companies also provide certificates and security services for large organisations, but what you're looking for is what VeriSign calls a 'digital ID' and Thawte calls a 'personal email certificate'. You can request a certificate from the company website.

When issuing your certificate, the CA verifies that you do indeed control the email address that you specify, thereby preventing somebody else from getting a certificate in your name. This makes it a form of digital identification. Higher-security certificates are also available, whereby you present yourself to a CA in person, and show identification such as a driver's licence or passport.

VeriSign charges a modest annual fee (currently US$15, and free trials are offered), whereas Thawte does not charge for personal certificates. However, in my opinion VeriSign's set up process is easier to use. On the other hand, Thawte provides an option of more sophisticated mechanisms for proving your identity.

Always bear in mind that certificates are ultimately based on trust, so you must use a CA that you are confident will guard your certificates and will be accepted by people with whom you exchange digital signatures.

Digitally signing email messages

To sign an email message digitally before sending it, select the menu or toolbar option to add a digital signature. Figure 13.2 shows the digital signature and encryption options as they appear in Thunderbird, Outlook Express 6 and Outlook 2002. For Outlook 2002, first select the **View → Options** menu item, then press the **Security Settings** button. Note that Netscape Mail's security features are similar to those of Mozilla Thunderbird's.

When you press **Send**, your mail application creates a digital signature from the message, using your private key, and appends this to the message. It also appends your digital certificate, containing your certified email address and your public key.

When the message is received, if the recipient's email application supports S/MIME it will use your public key to verify that the signature matches the message, to show that it has not been tampered with, and verify that it did in fact come from the correct email address, to show that it has not been forged. Some older or more rudimentary email clients are not S/MIME-compliant. However, they will still display the plain-text email message.

One final minor point here: a digital signature is completely different from a mail signature, which is a fixed block of text that you can set up to be appended to all messages, typically with your name and contact details.

Encrypting email messages

To send a colleague an encrypted email message, you will need to know what his or her public key is. The easiest way to get somebody's public key is to receive a digitally signed message from that person, as his or her digital certificate containing the key will be attached.

The options for encrypting messages are located alongside those for digitally signing them, as shown in Fig. 13.2. If you have not received that colleague's certificate or you have not stored it along with your email contacts, you will not be able to do this. But if you have, the process happens seamlessly. Your email application replaces the body of the mail message (not the subject, incidentally) with a version that is encrypted using the recipient's public key.

When the recipient receives it, the email application decrypts it automatically using the private key, and it is displayed like any other email message. Since the sender will have first sent you a digitally signed message, you can be confident that that person's email application supports the S/MIME security standard.

Operating system and internet security

This section discusses a range of issues related to the security of your computer's operating system (OS) and network. It discusses how to keep your OS up to date, how to make your internet access more secure, and

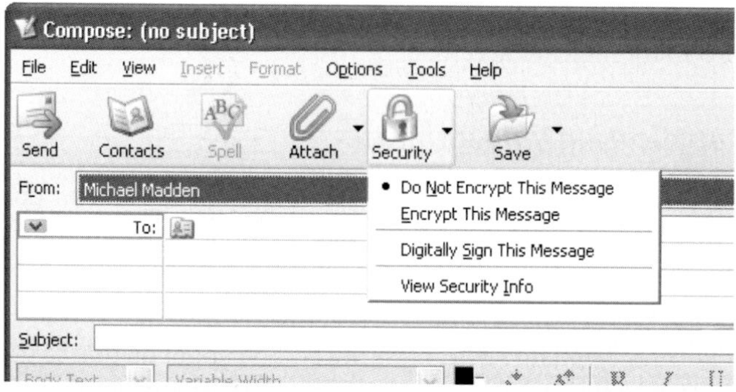

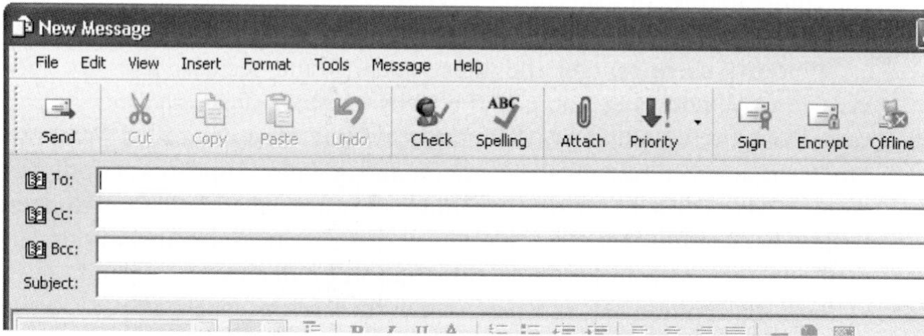

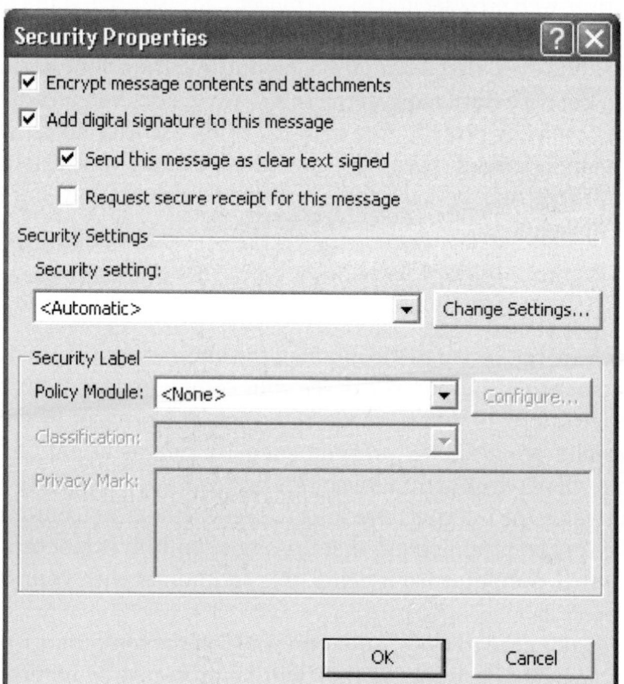

Fig. 13.2 The digital signature and encryption options as they appear in Thunderbird (top), Outlook Express (middle) and Outlook (bottom).

how to prevent computers for which you are responsible being used for inappropriate internet access.

OS and application vulnerabilities

No complex software system is completely bug free, and an operating system such as Windows, Linux or Mac OS X is a very complex software system. Since the OS is responsible for managing the interactions between all hardware, software, data and network connections, OS bugs can give rise to vulnerabilities that crackers may be able to discover and exploit to attack a computer. Computer worms, for example, principally spread by exploiting the vulnerabilities of a specific OS. When OS developers correct a bug, they release a system update, but it is up to you to install updates promptly.

Windows users can get the latest updates and security fixes for their version of Windows by going to the website *http://windowsupdate.microsoft.com*. Even better, Windows XP comes with a program called Windows Update that will automatically check for and download updates periodically. Apple's Mac OS X has a similar built-in feature called Software Updates under the **Apple** menu. Various Linux distributions also include update facilities; refer to your Linux documentation for details.

Bugs in applications that use network services, such as your email application, web browser and movie player, can also leave your computer vulnerable to attack. You should therefore keep all of your software updated.

Note, however, that I am talking about updating your *existing* software version, not necessarily upgrading to a new version. Vendors of commercial software typically provide free updates to fix security holes, whereas you have to buy upgrades. If you are comfortable using your existing software version, there may be no strong reason to upgrade, but you should still keep it updated.

Firewalls

Once you are connected to the internet, the internet is connected to you! This means that other computers can see your computer and attempt to connect to it. Such attempts may be made by computer worms or by crackers.

Firewalls are used to prevent such unwanted attention. A firewall monitors all network communications between your computer and external computers on the internet, checking to see whether they conform to specific criteria. Any communication that does not conform is blocked, preventing the external computer from being able to interact with your computer or even detect it.

You do not need to worry about firewalls on the computers in the hospital or clinic where you work, as they will be protected by enterprise firewall systems. The discussion here is relevant only to computers that have a direct connection to the internet, typically via a modem (dial-up or broadband).

There are two main categories of firewall: hardware-based and software-based. Software firewalls (or personal firewalls) use your computer's processor and could therefore potentially slow it down a little, but they are interactive so you can see warnings about potential intrusions and requests to allow communications.

A hardware firewall is a simple appliance that sits between your computer and the internet. ADSL modems (used for broadband internet access) and routers (used to connect computers together in your internal network) usually have built-in firewalls. They are not complicated to configure; refer to the manufacturer's documentation.

Good software firewall support is built into Linux, and Linux is used by many organisations on the servers that link all computers inside the organisation to the outside world. The Red Hat Linux distribution includes two tools for setting up a personal firewall: the Security Level Configuration Tool and GNOME Lokkit.

Mac OS X also includes a built-in personal firewall, or you can use a third-party firewall product. A popular shareware one is Brickhouse for OS X.

For Windows users, the two most often recommended software firewalls are ZoneAlarm (*http://www.zonelabs.com*) and Symantec's Norton Personal Firewall (*http://www.symantec.com/sabu/nis/npf*). The basic version of ZoneAlarm is free; there is also a 'Pro' version with additional security features beyond basic firewall functionality. Windows XP Pro includes quite a basic firewall, which is enabled by opening your **Network Connections** on the Control Panel, right clicking on a connection, selecting the **Properties** option, then going to the **Advanced** tab and pressing **Settings** to display the dialogue box shown in Fig. 13.3. Its main limitation is that it monitors incoming communications only. The only time you'll have unauthorised outgoing communications from your computer is when it is infected with a worm or Trojan, and good antivirus software provides an alternative defence against these. Given that third-party personal firewalls are inexpensive or free and offer good functionality, you should consider using one instead of XP's built-in one. However, bear in mind that you should never run two software firewalls simultaneously. Conversely, it is considered good practice to have both a hardware firewall and a software firewall.

Third-party firewall software products are, in general, easy to configure. They typically take a conservative approach, initially blocking all your applications from communicating across the internet, until you say otherwise. Therefore, for the first while after you install one it will display messages equivalent to the one from ZoneAlarm shown in Fig. 13.4. You will quickly discover that more applications use the internet than you thought! For example, some may check for updates and some may connect to the web for online help. You will also see some you don't recognise; these are likely to be OS services. Before answering yes or no, type the application name into a web search engine to find out about it.

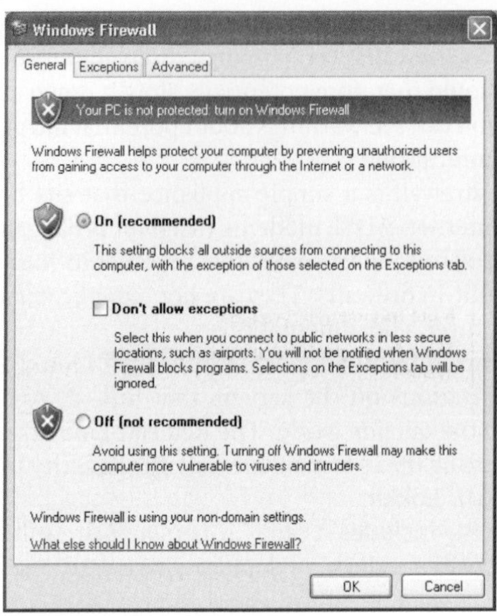

Fig. 13.3 Enabling Windows XP's built-in firewall.

To test your firewall, websites such as the McAfee-sponsored HackerWatch.org (*http://www.hackerwatch.org/probe/*) perform a scan of your computer and report what level of access external computers have to it. Other websites offering similar services are *http://scan.sygate.com* and Gibson Research at *http://grc.com/default.htm* (scroll down to find the link to ShieldsUP). You don't have to be using these manufacturers' products in order to use their firewall tests.

Wireless networks

Wireless local area networks (WLANs) based on the 802.11 standard are extremely popular, as they allow home and office users access to email, local area networks and the internet at up to 300 metres from the access point (AP). This is great from a user perspective, but terrible from a security perspective. Anybody with a laptop in a cafe down the street might be able to connect to your network and your computers. You may be able to secure your office physically, but you'll hardly be able to create a demilitarised zone of 300-metre radius around it. Therefore, there are a few basic steps to securing your WLAN's AP, listed next. Your AP will either come with special software for performing configuration or will have a web interface for doing so. Note that some APs are integrated into network routers, whereas others are separate boxes. Also, most routers also include built-in hardware firewalls.

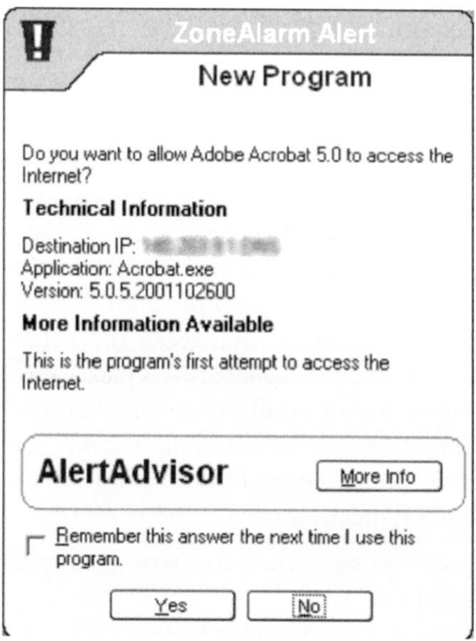
ZoneAlarm Alert
New Program
Do you want to allow Adobe Acrobat 5.0 to access the Internet?
Technical Information
Destination IP:
Application: Acrobat.exe
Version: 5.0.5.2001102600
More Information Available
This is the program's first attempt to access the Internet.
AlertAdvisor
More Info
Remember this answer the next time I use this program.
Yes
No

Fig. 13.4 A personal firewall verifying an application is legitimate.

Making your wireless AP/router more secure

- Change the default password and the default WLAN name.
- Don't use a WLAN name such as DR_SMITH_OFFICE that makes it easy for a snooper to know they've found you.
- Disable broadcasting of your WLAN's identifier (called its SSID), so that it will be difficult to find for computers that don't already know about it.
- Enable WEP (see below).
- Use MAC address filtering (a MAC address is a unique network identifier that every computer has). MAC filtering configures your router to accept connections only from computers with specific MAC addresses.

WEP (Wireless Encryption Protocol) works by using encryption when exchanging data between a computer and the AP. Unlike the public key encryption described above, it uses a single shared encryption key. This involves picking a random number with 26 hexadecimal digits (that is, in base 16, using digits 0–9 and letters A–F) and configuring the AP *and* all of your computers' wireless cards to use it. You must of course guard this number carefully.

Unfortunately, although WEP and MAC address filtering in theory provide good protection for your computers, in practice they can be compromised. That is why it is important to use all of the wireless security measures listed above.

Blocking access to inappropriate material

In your role as an employer or manager, you may be responsible for computers that other people use. (David Harris discusses the legal risks associated with this in Chapter 12.) Most employers address such issues through a combination of company policies, clear guidelines and employee education. However, there are circumstances in which you may also be interested in providing technological solutions to back up your policies.

A web content filter offers some protection. This is a program through which all web traffic is directed. It checks the origin and content of all material, and can prevent the display of web pages, either partially or fully.

Two well-known web content filters are NetNanny (*http://www.netnanny.com*) and SurfControl (*http://www.surfcontrol.com*); search on the web for 'web access filter' or 'web content filter' to find others.

Web access filters typically work on the basis of:

- blacklisted sites – those known to carry pornographic, racist or other offensive material
- whitelisted sites – those known to be legitimate
- blocked phrases
- content type – you may choose to block some categories but allow others.

The lists of blacklisted sites are usually maintained by the software providers, and the web access filter downloads revised lists frequently. You will typically specify whitelisted sites yourself, to avoid, for example, phrases being blocked when you read an online research journal that carries articles about the long-term effects of sexual violence. The software typically comes with a predefined dictionary of blocked phrases to which you can add or subtract. Current technology is not good enough to reliably inspect images themselves to determine whether they might be offensive, although research is ongoing.

Naturally, you should ensure before you use web/email filtering and monitoring software that it is legal to use for the purpose that you have in mind. Most of this software was originally designed to allow parents to monitor their children and employers to prevent employees from making unauthorised use of internet resources, but different rules may apply if users are not employees or if you monitor them without their knowledge.

File and folder security

This section discusses protection of files and folders, so that a cracker who accesses your computer physically or remotely will be unable to read sensitive files. As well as protecting your computer, it is particularly important to use the file encryption facilities supported by most USB drives, if you are storing sensitive patient information on one, as they are easily lost or stolen.

Document passwords

Some applications, such as Microsoft Word, Excel and Adobe Acrobat, allow you to password protect the documents they generate. In Microsoft Office applications, passwords are specified under the **Tools** → **Options** menu item, on the **Security** tab. This is a simple way of protecting your files, but is not a strong form of security.

A point to note is that Microsoft Office applications also support passwords that allow documents to be viewed but not modified. In a knowledge base article (*http://support.microsoft.com/default.aspx?scid=kb;en-us;822924*), Microsoft makes it clear that 'no modification' passwords do not offer security protection, and can be easily inspected and removed.

A high level of document security is provided by Adobe Acrobat 6, the 'official' software application for creating PDF documents. It includes functionality to digitally sign and encrypt PDF documents using digital certificates, as described earlier, providing authentication, non-repudiation and integrity. Acrobat's online help explains the steps.

File and folder encryption

Newer OSs support automatic encryption of folders and files, built into the file system. Windows XP Professional, for example, has Encrypting FileSystem built in, and Mac OS X has a similar built-in facility called FileVault. A number of filesystems supporting encryption have also been developed for Linux.

Using these facilities is easy. In Windows XP, for example, you simply right click on a file or folder and select **Properties**. Under the **General** tab, press the **Advanced** button to display the **Advanced Attributes** dialogue box. Simply ticking the **Encrypt** box encrypts the file. True to form, the procedure in Mac OS X is even simpler.

Files are encrypted and decrypted using public key cryptography. However, bear in mind that the purpose of this facility is to protect files while they are on the computer disk; if you copy the file to another disk that does not support encryption, or attach it to an email message, the copy is automatically decrypted.

Guard your digital certificates!

If you decide to use Windows XP's Encrypting FileSystem, it is essential that you spend a little time learning how to back up and protect the associated digital certificates. If they are deleted or lost in a hard drive crash, you will *never* be able to decrypt all your most valuable data. A helpful guide may be found at *http://www.practicalpc.co.uk/computing/windows/xpencrypt1.htm*.

Identity security

The topic of identity security conjures up images of elaborate ploys to take over a person's life by stealing or reproducing their credit cards, driver's licence and bank accounts. Identity theft such as this has been the subject of several Hollywood films. Here, however, we are concerned with simple techniques by which you might be persuaded by an impostor to divulge confidential information. An awareness of such techniques should help you guard against them.

Social engineering

Naive users can often be persuaded to give out passwords just by asking them. A classic trick is to contact a user by email or phone, claiming to be a systems administrator trying to track down a problem ('You'll probably have noticed that your outbound email is very slow this morning…') and simply to ask the person for username and password.

More elaborate versions of this technique, known as social engineering, involve contacting a user over the course of several days to establish credibility before requesting the password.

The technique has other applications. An impostor may attempt to acquire confidential patient information by establishing a persona as a health professional or researcher. Rather than contacting their targets by phone, impostors may use email or even written communications with official-looking headed paper, as indirect communications will allow him or her to formulate plausible responses to questions more easily.

What to watch out for

According to information provided by the Computer Security Institute (*http://www.gocsi.com*), some of the key signs that a person is engaging in social engineering are as follows:

- avoiding giving contact information
- rushed requests for information
- intimidation and name dropping
- asking odd questions
- minor mistakes (e.g. misspellings and misnomers)
- requests for confidential information.

If you consider the informal way in which we first make acquaintance with many of our trusted colleagues, it is clear that, with patience, an impostor may be able to insinuate himself or herself with us. This is a social issue rather than a technical one; the only solution is to be vigilant.

Personation

A related form of deception involves setting up an email account (or website) that looks like it belongs to somebody else. After all, there is nothing stopping you from signing up for an email account called *michael_g_madden@yahoo.co.uk*. You could even proceed to the VeriSign website and get a digital certificate to match!

You could then start sending email messages to my friends and colleagues, pretending to be me. While people might notice that my email address is different to usual, most people would not raise an eyebrow; many people have two or more email addresses.

Personators often pretend to be somebody that you do not know well, to make the job of imitating them easier. Like social engineering, the key is to be vigilant to unusual requests for information of a confidential nature, particularly if the requester is using a different email address from the standard work one. If in doubt, casually phone the person to clarify what exact information he or she needs. If the request did in fact come from a personator, you'll find out pretty quickly.

A related concept is 'phishing', where you receive a message asking you, for example, to update your online banking system details and directing you to a website that is a mock-up of the real bank one. Personal details that you enter are recorded and may be used later to steal money. Similar strategies are used to steal other forms of personal information.

Email spoofing

As was mentioned earlier, it is trivial to configure your mail client so that the 'from' field of your messages displays somebody else's email address. This is referred to as email spoofing. It can be used to make it seem as if the email came from someone you trust, in an attempt to persuade you to part with confidential information.

Email spoofing is of course related to personation; the difference here is that the email message will appear to come from the sender's usual address. As before, vigilance is most important. However, digital signatures can help. If a message is digitally signed, you can easily check whether the email address in the digital certificate matches the email address shown in the 'from' field.

Conclusions and security checklist

Unfortunately, it is impossible to make your computer completely secure; a sufficiently knowledgeable and determined cracker may be able to discover some avenue of access to your data. Therefore, protecting your computer's

Box 13.1 Security checklist

- If you work in a hospital or clinic, follow the institutional backup procedures
- Frequently back up the other computers for which you are responsible, using backup software with an automatic schedule
- Store backups and all other removable storage securely
- Follow the good practice for passwords
- Ensure all employees have different login accounts and are security aware
- Don't leave your computer unprotected by a password when unattended
- Supervise repair people or others to whom you give access to your data
- Digitally sign all of your email messages
- Encrypt sensitive messages
- Keep your software updated to protect against vulnerabilities
- For computers with direct internet connections, install and configure a hardware firewall and a personal software firewall
- Password protect shared folders and remove the share when not in use
- If you use a wireless network, follow the manufacturer's instructions for increasing its security
- Be aware of the issues in relation to access to inappropriate material from computers for which you are responsible
- Protect sensitive documents with passwords, or digital signatures and encryption if supported
- Consider using your operating system's support for folder encryption; if you do, make sure you know how to recover your data if your digital certificates are lost
- Be vigilant of impostors who may use social engineering, personation and email spoofing techniques to persuade to you release confidential information.

security requires multiple strategies. Many of these interact with each other. For example, if somebody gains physical access to your computer, and can figure out your password, he or she could send email messages with digital signatures that you would find very hard to repudiate.

The checklist in Box 13.1 summarises the main action points covered in this chapter. If you implement all of these, you can feel satisfied that you have made reasonable efforts to guard your data's security.

Suggested reading

Books

Alexander, M. (1996) *The Underground Guide to Computer Security*. London: Addison-Wesley. (Accessible but a little out-of date.)

Greene, T. C. (2004) *Computer Security for the Home and Small Office*. Berekely, CA: APress.

Russell, D. & Gangemi, G. T. (1991) Computer Security Basics. Sebastopol, CA: O'Reilly. (Mainly aimed at a corporate audience.)

Websites

Home Network Security, by CERT: *http://www.cert.org/tech_tips/home_networks.html* (Good overview for the general user.)

Home Computer Security, by CERT: *http://www.cert.org/homeusers/HomeComputerSecurity/* (Good overview for the general user.)

ITS-Med Information Security: *http://its.med.yale.edu/security/* (The website of Yale Medical School's Information Security Office, with information for doctors on good practice and policies.)

Security Documents: *http://www.SecurityDocs.com* (A comprehensive technical resource with white papers on many security topics.)

Security-related news and articles: *http://www.theregister.co.uk/security/* (Interesting and accessible topical articles.)

CHAPTER 14

Clinical information systems and the psychiatrist

Martin Elphick and Matt Evans

The previous chapters of this book have mostly concentrated on general-purpose computer software. But over the next decade we can expect to see specialist health information systems becoming available, even in mental health units, at least in affluent countries. Just as supermarket workers operate their tills with no understanding of the underlying technology, mental health staff should be able to carry out a range of common tasks with very little training.

All of these systems, whatever the size, are founded on principles that are easy for a clinician to understand, and which we will describe in this chapter. There is, unfortunately, space to give only an overview of these important topics but we intend to guide readers towards the most relevant information. In particular, we aim to show how they may play an important role in managing clinical information systems within their workplace.

The evolution of health information systems

Over the years some of the most successful clinical systems have developed from simple local software programs written by clinicians into commercial products. However, with such a patchwork of different systems in use, information sharing was impeded and staff had to learn to use each application anew.

The ambitious 'National Programme for IT' for England (NPfIT, presently called 'NHS Connecting for Health') is the biggest single investment in information technology (IT) of any type attempted in the world. It includes a 10-year plan to create a comprehensive 'national care record', which will allow patients to be treated in any setting, with the health professional able to access any necessary clinical information immediately. It is likely that the rest of the UK (and perhaps other countries worldwide) will take a similar path. Indeed, international work on creating standards for health care records has been going on for many years (examples include: the Good European Health Record, *http://www.chime.ucl.ac.uk/work-areas/ehrs/GEHR/*; European Standard ENV13606, *http://www.centc251.org*; Health Level 7, *http://www.hl7.org*; and Open HER, *http://www.openehr.org*).

Most health professionals have a general idea of the benefits of clinical information systems and welcome their arrival. For others, though, the prospect of computers intruding on clinical life is undesirable, daunting or even terrifying.

We can't expect systems to be installed without investing considerable resources in educating and training the users. This starts with basic computing skills (some of which are covered in this book) and the opportunity for users to develop their confidence. For most clinicians this will include web browsing, email, word processing and presentation software. Training will then need to be provided on the specific clinical information system in use. Beyond this, though, it is important in this information age for all psychiatrists to develop information management skills and have a basic understanding of 'health informatics' (see below). This will become an increasingly important training requirement and a feature of continuing professional development (CPD).

Components of a health information system

Imagine a set of paper notes without dividers between the sections. It would be a bit of a mess and rather hard to use. When we move to an electronic record we must be equally well organised and structured in our approach. The precise structure of our care record will depend on what systems we are using. It is likely, however, that the record will be stored across many separate sub-systems, probably in different physical locations, and that it will be pulled together only when we access it through the user interface. This section provides a simplified description of this process.

The patient record

This is perhaps the hardest element of a health information system to define. It is what most people think of as the computerised record. It has been known at various times by names such as electronic patient record (EPR), electronic care record (ECR), electronic health record (EHR), electronic health care record (EHCR) and integrated mental health electronic record (IMHER). In addition to the basic 'clinical notes' it may also contain additional functions and information (discussed further below). The way the clinical information is entered and exchanged is very important and this is described in the section on standards.

Patient administration/demographics system

All health information systems require, at their core, a system to manage patient demographic details. The generic name for this is patient administration system (PAS) and it may be built into some patient records or act as a separate server-based database. Every patient must have a unique identity so that all other systems can be certain they are dealing with the same patient.

The front end

Even consumer-level software is very complex, but the powerful 'enterprise' systems we are discussing are even more so. The art of the 'user interface' designer is to create 'front ends' (the bit you interact with) which hide this complexity while enabling staff to use the system with confidence.

Access to these systems must be rapid if it is to be useful in a clinical setting, particularly during emergencies. After entering a password and typing a few letters of the patient's name, the records of that individual should appear on-screen. The options available should reflect the tasks you are undertaking. By selecting these items it should be possible to access previously entered care information, review appointments, add new data or notes (perhaps using a word processing function), communicate with other clinicians, carers, or the patient (using email or messaging technology), prescribe, view protocols and guidelines, and so on. The system should be designed to support the way a psychiatrist works and should, to some extent, be customisable to match the local model of care.

Considerations specific to mental health

The Care Programme Approach (CPA) and Mental Health Act activity are areas of functionality specific to mental health but, for the most part, the functions of mental health systems are part of generic health systems or at least customisations of them. This does not mean, though, that any generic system is sufficiently customisable to meet the needs of psychiatrists. The working day of a mental health professional is very different from that of a colleague in, say, medicine or surgery and our systems need to support our mode of working. In addition, psychiatrists tend to write a great deal more than other doctors and this needs consideration when designing systems.

Decision support systems

These systems, as the name implies, are not intended to 'automate' healthcare or to remove clinical experience from decision making. Rather, they are designed to assist in making healthcare safer and more consistent, and to provide useful information when required. The simplest form might be to provide immediate access to online protocols. It might also take the form of a computerised 'care pathway' that can be invoked if certain criteria are met. An electronic care pathway can drive standardised care and generate suggested work lists for mental health professionals. It can help to ensure, for example, that all new admissions have a physical examination within 24 hours or that a urine drug screen is completed as per hospital policy. This type of automation is governed by what are often referred to as 'rules and alerts'. When certain conditions are met, an alert is raised to the relevant person; if no response is received, the next most senior person is alerted.

More complex decision support systems can be integrated with the clinical information itself to support diagnosis and treatment decisions directly.

Electronic prescribing

So-called e-prescribing has been shown to be of great benefit to patient safety (Audit Commission, 2001). Such systems may incorporate information on allergies and sensitivities as well as prescribing records. A single drug record shared across hospital, community and general practice should eliminate errors that occur through poor communication. Similarly, integration with decision support should provide error checks and prescribing advice.

Pathology systems and orders

The majority of hospitals already run pathology systems in which results can be reviewed on the hospital network. In future, most requests will also be computerised. The general term for this process is 'orders'. Blood tests, radiographs, urine testing, physiotherapy assessment, medication and even a Mini Mental State Examination could be 'ordered' in this way. Radiology systems will run picture archiving and communications systems (PACS), which allow radiology images such as computerised tomography scans to be viewed remotely on the computer screen.

Service user involvement

The new systems offer the chance to involve service users in many aspects of their care, including having their own space within their record so they can contribute to it. This might be to record how they feel, to complete a Beck Depression Inventory on a weekly basis or to keep a diary during a course of cognitive–behavioural therapy. They might also flag up inaccuracies in their record. Service users are likely to have their own screens on which to view their record during ward rounds or CPA meetings. A further benefit to service users is the ability to book and rearrange appointments online.

Staff directory

In the same way that a patient administration system is required to list every patient, there is also a need to identify every staff member uniquely within an organisation, no matter what its size. Each entry in the notes must be assigned to a known individual and it must be possible to contact that individual at a later date. Once registered on a system-wide directory, a health professional will be able to move between hospitals and still be recognised. It follows that in systems covering large areas, an electronic register or directory of clinical teams or services (each with its own unique identity) will also be required in order to provide 'addresses' for communications, and to assign a role to each health professional.

At the coal face

Multi-agency care, and the care journey sequence

A trend in mental health information systems has been evolution towards 'integrated' systems that support multi-agency collaborative care. Systems now aim to provide the full range of functions that are necessary at each stage of the patient's care journey. It will be possible to receive electronic referrals, look up past notes, book a date for an assessment interview, let everyone know what you are about to do, fill in a standard assessment form (in collaboration with other agencies and using third-party information if necessary), distribute it, make an electronic prescription that will go straight to the pharmacy and general practitioner, notify anyone who needs to know about risks, and so on, until discharge. This sharing could occur across all members of the multidisciplinary team (including social workers, occupational therapists and community psychiatric nurses) so long as they have a 'legitimate relationship' with the patient. Each time an 'event' such as face-to-face or telephone contact, assessment, admission or discharge is entered, this can be registered for management purposes.

The record kept by such a system is sequential, in the sense that successive entries can potentially be read in the order of the events that they refer to, as well as the order in which they were entered into the computer. A note can be 'slotted in' after the event, and if a wrong entry is made for any reason, it can be modified later. The virtual sequential nature of the record is an essential part of its organisation.

Electronic CPA

With all of this potential for information recording and instant multi-agency communications, will the new technology make the CPA unnecessary? It will certainly replace some aspects. The benefits to the service user, though, of bringing together the relevant care professionals for a meeting (even in a virtual sense) cannot be overstated. An agreement between people on the essential points of each assessment and care plan will still need to be reached from time to time, and those decisions will need to be entered as a record at that specific date.

It is easy to get confused as to what might happen after that. Just as is the case with paper records, each piece of information in the CPA summary may subsequently change and other parts of the record will need to be updated accordingly. But the CPA summary itself will have to remain unchanged until the next review is authorised by the care coordinator. A CPA summary, in other words, cannot function both as a reliable 'real time' summary of current care and as a summary of what was intended at some point in the past (as has been tacitly assumed for many years).

Information for managing services

Just as the clinician's pet computer programs did not tell the finance director very much that he or she needed to know, the patient administration system that the director commissioned tended not to help much with care plans, or getting the latest research information off the internet. For a long time clinical and management applications have run in parallel in this fashion. It was often repeated in policy documents that management information should be derived from data collected for clinical purposes. Only recently has there been real progress in this direction and in a few years it should no longer be necessary for clinicians to feed systems with specially collected data, from which no useful analysis or communication ever seems to emerge. Psychiatrists are in a unique position to motivate these improvements – after all, without psychiatrists the management data could not be collected.

As psychiatrists, we should be prepared to assist in the interpretation and critical appraisal of management information, since we are well placed to understand the environment from which it is derived, have training in statistics and research design, and have a personal stake in the results.

In a state health service like the NHS, managers (general and clinical) are there to make sure that enough clinicians are available in the right places and with sufficient resources to meet the population's health needs – according to priorities set democratically. In private care, priorities are set differently but the tasks are similar in many respects. Managers therefore need a top-down policy to guide them, information on local needs, and care data on which staff treated which patients, where, how often, with what intervention, for how long, and with what effect.

This information, which forms the basis of all 'reporting data-sets' (or 'minimum data-sets'), must be collected by clinicians and be anonymised and aggregated for various uses at different organisational levels:

- At team level, case-load management and clinical audit will be common uses.
- At intermediate levels contracts and service agreements will need to be set and monitored for volumes of activity, and for the type of cases being treated with particular interventions (case mix). Clinical governance also depends upon the availability of the right types of good-quality data – activity, case mix and intervention mix, and outcome.
- At the highest levels, public health statistics are needed to assess morbidity geographically, and the government will be attempting to assess how policy changes are coming into effect. 'Performance indicators' may be used for that purpose, although to date these have tended, out of necessity, to measure whatever can be measured, rather than the value of mental healthcare provision, which is hard to quantify.

Ideally, from the data listed above, managers should be able to work out the best distribution of money and resources and the cost-effectiveness of this distribution. None the less, there are numerous pitfalls in the use of such data. Data quality is often poor, owing to incomplete or erroneous entries, and the necessary cleaning of the data-set may introduce systematic errors. When data are analysed in sub-sets, invalid groupings are often used that lump dissimilar data together, causing what is sometimes called a 'perverse incentive' for healthcare providers to pay greater heed to some types of patients than others. For instance, by analysing all patients with ICD–10 affective disorders together in a service agreement, a provider will be paid the same for occasional supportive out-patient treatment of someone with dysthymia as for an in-patient episode for treatment-resistant mania. To get around these technical problems, 'case-mix groupings' are in development, which should include both the condition and the intervention used. This may in time provide the information required to deliver 'payment by results' in mental health services.

Psychiatrists should consider using the same principles in this sort of work that they would apply to a research project. In a well-designed trial, the same parameters as those listed above are deliberately restricted so that a specified hypothesis can be examined about the relationship between two variables (often the intervention and the outcome). In collecting routine data for management, audit and clinical governance purposes, the only difference is that we first collect all the types of data about all the patients in case we might need it and then subsequently use subsets of the data to test a variety of hypotheses. For instance, we could examine the outcomes of all patients with the same diagnosis treated by the same team, and it may be sufficient simply to know that the results are satisfactory.

Alternatively, we could compare their outcomes with those of similar patients treated by other teams, or against a national or regional benchmark. To do so with validity we must either analyse only patients treated with the same intervention for the same time and so on, or separately examine the effect of other variables that might affect outcome. If there seemed to be a difference, we could then generate secondary hypotheses to test, using the same data.

Note that this is different to scanning the data to see if there is anything that looks interesting, and then making up a retrospective hypothesis. Statistical tests of significance are rarely used in this field, but their potential validity should always be considered. While it is worth knowing how confident you can be in your results, routinely gathered information will more often be descriptive than comparative.

As a method of resource allocation this evidence-based approach contrasts sharply with the manipulation, histrionics and similar territorial behaviour that presently characterise the process.

Whether such 'management' activity is carried out by a senior clinician or a general manager will depend on local custom, but it seems a good thing for a psychiatrist at least to be able to follow the process, and to request or make relevant analyses of his or her own; and contribute to the debate. A good information system should allow for easy analyses by anyone with authority to do so. It should also be supported by good graphics.

Confidentiality and security

David Harris and Mike Madden have covered legal and security concerns comprehensively in Chapters 12 and 13 respectively. The Royal College of Psychiatrists has produced a Council report (CR85, January 2000) entitled *Good Practice Guidance on Confidentiality*, which is available on the College website (*http://www.rcpsych.ac.uk/publications/cr/cr85.htm*). However, it is worth reiterating the need for backups and redundancy in such a critical health infrastructure. In addition, audit facilities are vital so that those making entries and amendments to the system can be identified later if necessary. In most circumstances changes to the record should be visible to all.

The need for standards

Clinical records structures

The information we hold about a patient is useful not just within our own mental health service. For information to be truly transferable, it needs to conform to standards and it needs to be reusable across a range of settings. This is addressed in the plans for the English Care Record Service by means of the concept of 'care record elements' (CREs). An 'element' is a single piece of defined information, such as a differential diagnosis or a lithium level. A hierarchical structure to the CREs defines what clinical information belongs in what section. At the time of writing, the structure is being defined but it is likely to include major categories such as problems, diagnoses, findings and plans. Within these, the elements can be further divided, so that 'pathology results' will be found under 'findings'.

With standard, coded definitions for each element, the elements can be incorporated into clinical documents in whatever order or degree of complexity suits the clinical need. The development of documentation is therefore free from the constraints of any system of standard headings. Agreement on the headings across psychiatry or mental health services as a whole will come about through national and regional bodies and they will not need to be compromised to fit with the needs of a surgical clerking, for instance. The local mental health document will be a collection of elements juggled around to fit the needs of the mental health event. The English care record approach is just one way of tackling this and alternative approaches can be found in other work across the globe (such as Open HER, mentioned at the start of the chapter).

Clinical coding standards

Consider a diagnosis element referring to 'cord compression' in a female patient. A human would infer from the context (here, being under the care of an obstetrician) that it was the umbilical cord being compressed. A computer, however, lacks this contextualising ability and could easily decide that a neurosurgical emergency was imminent. Similar confusion could arise from the term 'sectioned' referring as it does to tissue preparations, operative intervention in childbirth and the use of the Mental Health Act.

Such problems arise because the information is recorded as 'free text', which allows rich expression at the expense of computer interpretation. While the use of free text will remain necessary in many circumstances, it is better to use defined terms when the situation permits. Some systems permit free text to be appended to coded data to expand the meaning, giving the best of both worlds. Future systems will greatly enhance our ability to code work quickly from the free text we enter. Diagnosis is important to code but we really do not need to code all (or even most) of what we do.

Examples of current clinical coding schemes include the Read codes used by general practitioners and the SNOMED system used in the USA. Collaboration has resulted in SNOMED CT, which will become the NHS coding standard. A basic knowledge of it will be required of all psychiatrists, although mostly it will run unseen in the background of many clinical systems.

Health informatics

Health informatics (HI) is the academic discipline that studies the use of information, communications and technology to bring about improvements in healthcare. In the work setting, health informatics (sometimes shortened to informatics) is about analysing the way in which healthcare organisations (such as a mental health trust) operate in terms of information flows, user interactions and so on, and then developing and implementing solutions.

Table 14.1 A selection of postgraduate health informatics courses

Institution	Course website
CHIME, University College London	http://www.chime.ucl.ac.uk/prospective-students/graduate-study/health-informatics-msc/index.htm
City University, London	http://www.soi.city.ac.uk/pgcourses/hi/
Coventry University	http://www.coventry.ac.uk/courses/course-a-z/a/628
Trinity College, Dublin	https://www.cs.tcd.ie/courses/mschi/
University of Bath/Royal College of Surgeons Edinburgh	http://www.health-informatics.info/
University of Central Lancashire	http://www.uclan.ac.uk/courses/depts/lshpm.htm
University College Winchester	http://www.wkac.ac.uk/Home.aspx?Page=3028
University of Leeds	http://www.ychi.leeds.ac.uk/content/2300.aspx?cat=MSC
University of Sheffield	http://www.shef.ac.uk/is/courses/pg_mschi.html
University of Wales, Swansea	http://www.ihi.aber.ac.uk/MSc.asp
University of Warwick	http://www2.warwick.ac.uk/study/postgraduate/medicine/his/
University of the West of England	http://info.uwe.ac.uk/courses/viewcourse.asp?urn=10007

Health informatics is as diverse as medicine itself and the evidence base for what we are doing is ever growing. Many of the basic principles have been mentioned throughout this chapter and they will increasingly become incorporated in professional training and job descriptions. For those with a strong interest (especially if you intend to develop your career along these lines), you are advised to consider taking one of several diploma or MSc courses that run in the UK (see Table 14.1).

The psychiatrist's role in developing and implementing health information systems

Throughout this chapter, we have tried to incorporate clinical examples of how the new mental health information systems will affect us all. Traditionally, psychiatrists may have had a role in developing (even coding!) systems within their hospital. They may have sat on committees developing local strategy, allocating funds and choosing hardware.

Our feeling is that, within the UK at least, this situation is likely to change somewhat, because of the huge national procurements now in train. There are now even more opportunities than ever to get involved though. At national level, there are structures in place to ensure widespread stakeholder consultation (with clinicians, managers, patients, carers, medical

Royal Colleges etc.). In addition, those with specialist informatics skills are involved in designing and planning the new systems. It is possible to be involved at this level but it is probably best to get involved initially at local or regional level.

Within the English procurement clusters there are local clinical design and implementation groups that are responsible for recommending system design on evidence-based or best-practice lines. They have a mix of practising mental health clinicians from across the region and meet regularly. They work to ensure that the systems will not just support national standards but also meet the specific requirements of the local services they represent. It is a good idea to find out who is representing your area and to maintain communication with these people. You will then have a good idea of what is happening nationally and regionally, as well as being able to feed in ideas from your local service.

At local level, our experience is that rather than trying to tackle issues from an 'IT perspective', the better approach is to incorporate informatics in all that we do. Clinical governance, audit and general service improvement are highly reliant on informatics. Journal clubs and grand rounds can be enriched by consideration of how information systems affect clinical care.

Psychiatrists are in an ideal position to take an active local role in the process of implementing systems and managing the change process. It is advisable to appoint clinical leads (multiprofessional, not just psychiatrists) and they can advise on how best to address local issues. Suggested areas include:

- surveying local computer skills
- planning training requirements
- supervising the review of data quality for returns
- generating ideas exciting to psychiatrists
- easing the pains of the change process
- communicating national and regional strategies to other clinicians
- liaising with local IT services
- taking part in pilot studies
- reviewing care pathways and protocols for implementation
- deciding on the customisation of rules and alerts
- standardising clinical documentation
- monitoring the effect of computer use on therapeutic relationships
- supervising trainees in informatics.

Such a workload is likely to require some protected sessions but the role is far too important to ignore.

Further reading

Audit Commission (2001) *A Spoonful of Sugar – Medicines Management in NHS Hospitals.* London: Audit Commission.

CHAPTER 15

Future developments

Bruce Taylor

The perils of prognostication

Since many of the topics discussed in this chapter will seem somewhat science fictional, it might be appropriate to open with a mention of an old SF story in which a grizzled asteroid miner calculates a trajectory for his spaceship using ... a slide rule. In the 1950s, privately owned spaceships obviously seemed a realistic prediction but a privately owned computer was too much even for a science-fiction writer. Now, of course, we predict a future filled with computers and networks, perhaps not realising that the dominant technology of tomorrow might be based on some currently obscure area of knowledge like colloid chemistry. However, the SF writer was brave enough to nail his colours to the mast and so shall I. It is my prediction that computers and information technology in the broadest sense will be an increasingly important force in the shaping of tomorrow's mental health services.

In this chapter I will first look at some plausible future technologies, before moving on to an examination of how these technologies might affect our lives at work and at home over the next few years.

The technologies themselves

Improvements in networking

The most obvious improvement is in the speed and capacity of network connections. For those of us who remember the expensive and slow dial-up connections of the early to mid-1990s, a modern broadband connection is nothing short of miraculous. Most home users subscribe to ADSL (asymmetric digital subscriber line – what most people would understand as 'broadband' currently – which is asymmetric because the download speed is substantially faster than the upload speed), but DSL (digital subscriber line) is also available to home users. Symmetric connections such as DSL, perhaps using fibre optics, may be more common in a 'peer to peer' future in which both upload and download speed will be valued.

This increase in speed has been accompanied by an increase in pervasiveness, particularly by the use of wireless technology to extend the network. The advertising stereotypes for this change include the home worker checking work email in the garden or the harried executive who sees his child's first smile on the screen of a videophone.

The clinical applications of fast, ubiquitous networking go far beyond these marketing clichés, however. The challenge for today's National Health Service (NHS) is to deliver quality clinical care to a demanding public under tight budgetary scrutiny. It is easy to see how the ability to access relevant information rapidly at the point of care could help support these objectives.

Network applications

Email

Email is one of the earliest, and is still one of the most popular, network applications. When the basic email protocols were laid down, the internet was a smaller and more trusting place, so security and authentication were not high priorities. This, along with a lack of security at the level of both the application and the operating system (OS), has led to the incredible situation where the majority of email traffic is spam, much of it infested with malicious software. There are active efforts by industry and standards bodies to rectify these deficiencies and deliver a secure and trustworthy email infrastructure.

If these efforts succeed, we can hope that email will not only return to its former glory but also take over functions that are currently served by paper mail, such as confidential communication or authenticated delivery.

The asynchronous nature of email has always been one of its best features, as it permits communication without interruption. Email is also easily integrated into calendar, contacts and to-do applications such as Microsoft's Outlook program or IBM's Lotus Notes. In the future, we will probably see further developments in the integration of email into other software.

Telephony

It is likely that the present stampede away from landlines and towards mobile phones will continue. Indeed, some developing countries have leapfrogged the landline stage entirely and moved straight to digital mobile networks.

Now that telephone calls, whether from a fixed or mobile handset, have gone digital there is a strong rationale for treating them as just another form of network service, by routing them over the same networks used for web browsing, email and instant messaging. Such 'voice over IP' (VOIP) systems are becoming popular with price-conscious consumers and businesses alike. The popular Skype service (*http://www.skype.com*) is one provider of VOIP.

Future telephones therefore are likely to be very smart devices, with the ability to choose the best connection method depending on location, and able to support a variety of functions such as file transfer, email, instant messaging and web browsing, as well as VOIP. Many of these features can be seen in embryonic form in the smartphones discussed in Chapter 9.

Instant messaging

Instant messaging (or IM) has long been popular with those computer users who enjoyed permanent network connections. Examples include the internet relay chat (IRC) system, ICQ, AIM or Yahoo chat. Messages are typed into and read from a small window on-screen in a way that is more akin to a conversation than an email. With the increased availability of permanent network connections, this kind of application will probably increase in popularity and may merge with the SMS (text) message system on mobile phones.

Instant messaging is also under consideration for computer–computer or computer–human communication. Even today, there are IRC 'bots' (software programs) that can sustain a realistic conversation, at least for a short time. A more advanced version of such a program could, conceivably, be part of your calendar or to-do system, providing discreet reminders of appointments, tasks and messages, and answering simple queries on your behalf. See *http://smarterchild.conversagent.com* for an early prototype of such a system.

Videoconferencing

Telemedicine has been defined by Ian McClelland as the 'use of telecommunications to improve clinical diagnosis, care, and efficiency'. Telepsychiatric videoconferencing began in 1961 with the successful use of a two-way analogue television link in group therapy.

As with telemedicine generally, the development of inexpensive digital communication technology in the 1990s increased the pace of telepsychiatry research. According to Yellowlees, psychiatry has taken the lead among medical specialties in promoting remote consultation.

Does it mean, however, that those living in areas served by telepsychiatry are receiving a second-rate service? The available evidence suggests that this is not the case. In a study involving 10 patients with obsessive–compulsive disorder, Baer and colleagues found no significant difference in inter-rater reliabilities between local and telepsychiatric raters on several scales. They also found that the telepsychiatric system was acceptable to the participants, a finding replicated by other investigators.

A systematic review of the general telemedicine literature by Roine and his colleagues in 2001 concluded that telepsychiatry was one of the telemedicine applications for which 'the most convincing published evidence exists'.

File sharing

File sharing is the magic that you use at work to make hard disks on a hospital network server appear to be attached to whatever machine you are currently using. Thus, you can log on from the ward or in your office and be confident that you can still access your files (if you have been careful to save the files to the network drive in the first place). In addition, as Mike Madden explained in Chapter 13, a file server makes a fine backup device.

This kind of file sharing works best over a fast local network such as you might find in a workplace. It requires a centralised server with professional administrators. Until recently, small and home users were denied the benefits of these technologies. However, the increased take-up of broadband connections has now created a market for web-based file storage facilities, essentially remote file servers owned by a specialist organisation. In addition, there have emerged several networks that offer file sharing without any centralised servers, so-called 'peer to peer' (P2P) systems like Freenet and Gnutella. This technology is often equated with copyright infringement and other dubious activities and it is true that a wide variety of illicit material is traded on some P2P networks. However, these systems also offer a glimpse of a future of truly distributed storage, where you will be able to access your information, suitably encrypted, anywhere in the world that you happen to be.

The web

For most people the web *is* the internet. However, from the preceding paragraphs it can be seen that the web is just one kind of application that can be run on top of a TCP/IP network (i.e. an intranet or the internet). The web as we know it was developed in the early 1990s in a physics research centre as a simple way of sharing information. The rapid adoption of the web was probably due to two factors: the relative simplicity of the protocols; and the absence of any intellectual property encumbrances on them.

The web has come a long way since the early days and now supports functions undreamt of by its creators. However, one of those creators, Sir Tim Berners-Lee, has been thinking about how his creation might be extended and he has concluded that what the present web lacks is any sense of *meaning*. For example, imagine using a search engine to look for 'apple'. Today's search engines have no way of knowing if you are interested in crunchy fruit, stylish computers or a theological discourse on original sin. The so-called semantic web would use what are called 'ontology servers', in addition to our familiar web servers. These specialised servers would contain definitions of what terms mean, their relationships to other terms and the inference rules by which conclusions could be drawn from these terms. The semantic web, or similar technology, would allow quite simple and unintelligent programs to perform some quite sophisticated reasoning, allowing more delegation of tasks to computers and reducing the time needed to find relevant information. For more on the semantic web see *http://www.sciam.com/article.cfm?articleID=00048144-10D2-1C70-84A9809EC588EF21&ref=sciam.*

Hardware developments

Input and output devices

Pen and paper scores over keyboards in those situations, common in medicine, when there is a need for data entry 'on the hoof'. There have, though, been personal digital assistants (PDAs – see Chapter 9) on which you write for some time now. Generally, these simplify the recognition task by requiring the user to learn a modified block alphabet. Recent PDA models and the larger tablet PCs have more sophisticated recognition that can cope with natural handwriting.

There are also signs of progress at the other, output end of the equation. We are currently in the middle of a transition from cathode-ray tube displays to liquid crystal displays (LCDs), which consume less power and space. Advances now making their way out of the laboratory include thin, flexible, paper-like displays that can be produced cheaply, that roll up for storage and that consume little power in use.

Another option that has found favour in specialist applications is the so-called head-up display (HUD). Derived from military flying equipment these displays project images and text over the user's normal field of vision at apparent visual infinity. This rather hallucinatory mixture of the real and the virtual world is referred to as 'augmented reality' and there are clear benefits in some medical specialties (think of a surgeon having the radiological images overlain on the real anatomy of the patient). The benefits to psychiatrists seem rather less and their use by clients will doubtless lead to a lot of phenomenological confusion!

Other hardware

We discussed hard disk drives in Chapter 1. These remain the mainstay of data storage, despite challenges from flash memory and other solid-state technologies (those with no moving parts).

Regardless of the underlying technology, it is possible that storage devices will themselves become smarter and more independent, capable of managing connections and disconnections to different computers and networks. Such a 'personal server' is available in concept form from Intel. Portable music players/hard drives such as the iPod represent another trend in the same direction.

If you link such a personal server with a head-up display using short-range wireless networking (Bluetooth) and a smartphone you have created a wearable computer. This rather Borg-like device is, according to some commentators, the next step beyond laptops and PDAs. While one might doubt the mass appeal of the current, rather nerdish models, this is nothing that could not be fixed with the application of some design expertise.

Many of us already have several chargers in our homes and cars to keep all of our gadgetry topped up. If these technologies are to be fully exploited, we will need something better than the current generation of lithium-ion batteries. Developments like fuel cells and exotic technologies like carbon nanotubes promise to meet this need.

Radio frequency identification devices (RFIDs) are touted as the answer to problems as diverse as tagging pets, managing inventories and enhancing medication concordance. In essence, these devices are very small chips, about the size of a grain of sand. They respond electronically when a scanner is passed over them, allowing, for example, a person to find out the contents of a box without opening it. The system is obviously useful in logistics as a replacement for bar codes. The chips can also be inserted into a pillbox or even individual pills as an aid to monitoring concordance. The obvious civil liberty implications of this will be discussed below.

Software developments

Recognition software

We discussed new input techniques above. Another approach to the same problem is to improve the ability of computers to recognise handwriting or speech rather than forcing humans to change their work habits. It is probably fair to say that, as a group, psychiatrists are not the most technophilic of doctors, so any improvements here would most likely be of great benefit.

There are commercially available packages for recognising both speech and handwriting, and while these are not yet a challenge to the supremacy of the keyboard, they may ease the transition to computerised systems for some users. In the future, we may yet return to simple pads of paper and dictation, but with clever software ensuring that our notes and letters are appropriately transcribed and filed.

Artificial intelligence

The term 'artificial intelligence' (or AI) means different things to different people. The creation of so-called 'strong' AI – conscious machines of human or superhuman intelligence – would result in an 'all bets off' situation, what the writer Vernor Vinge called the 'Singularity'. Making predictions about such an event is beyond the scope of this chapter.

More interesting from a predictive point of view is the prospect of computer systems able functionally to emulate some aspect of human cognition, so-called 'weak' AI. In the past, such systems were based on the idea (similar to cognitive psychology) that human intelligence is essentially like a series of algorithms (like life support training or the Maudsley rapid tranquillisation protocol) that could be captured in the form of rule sets and embodied in a computer program. While this approach has had some success (the 'wizard' that guides you through installing a new printer would be one example), overall it has proved a disappointment.

More recently, there have been developments in approaches that do not follow this rule-based approach but use instead looser, more 'subconscious' approaches to problem solving. Examples of this include neural networks, which are electronic components (or computer simulations of the same) arranged in a way loosely analogous to animal neurons and which are 'trained' rather than programmed to perform various tasks.

Another approach, again inspired by a biological metaphor, is genetic programming (see *http://www.genetic-programming.org*), in which the solution to a problem (often a problem in software design) is evolved over many generations by a process of variation and selection similar to the workings of biological evolution.

Other promising techniques fall under the rubric of 'pattern recognition'. For example, there exists software that can identify the abnormal (in a statistical sense) behaviour patterns that often precede a suicide on underground railway systems. The developers have also mentioned the possibility of applying the system to detecting falls or illness among elderly people living alone. (For further details see *http://www.newscientist.com/news/news.jsp?id=ns99993918*).

What is interesting about many of these applications is that, unlike conventional AI, the system does not embody an explicit model of the phenomena it tries to predict or recognise. Professionals employing such systems might be placed in an unusual situation if they were asked to justify a particular course of action. For example, a neural network might suggest, based on the processing of an enormous data-set, that certain, apparently irrelevant, behavioural or historical features were predictive of reoffending in a forensic population. Should this finding be included in risk assessment? Could such a risk assessment survive judicial scrutiny?

We have already mentioned the links between cognitive psychology and AI and between experimental neuroscience and neural network research. These links run in both directions, with computer science acting as a rich source of models for the behavioural sciences. This work has been engagingly summarised by writers such as Steven Pinker. Whether or not you agree with their materialist perspective, it is likely that the future will see further developments along these lines.

The remembrance agent

The convergence of clever software, massive storage, cheap cameras and wearable computers carried to its logical conclusion leads to the idea of recording and indexing one's entire life. Everything you see and hear, every face you see (linked to an address book) and place you go (tied into GPS coordinates), every email you send or receive and every document you work on would be filed away for future reference. This sounds impossibly ambitious but the amount of storage involved is actually relatively modest, in the order of one terabyte (1024 gigabytes) per year, according to Jim Gemmell and Gordon Bell of Microsoft, who are working on one version of this concept (see *http://research.microsoft.com/barc/mediapresence/MyLifeBits.aspx*). The clinical applications of such a system could include a form of 'memory prosthesis' for those in the early stages of dementia, as described in research from the University of Oregon (see *http://www.cs.uoregon.edu/research/wearables/projects.html*).

The electronic patient record

Some of the current work in this area was described in Chapter 14. The advanced electronic patient record (EPR) of the next few decades may combine the core record-keeping functionality with a degree of in-built intelligence, perhaps scanning the record for errors or suggesting relevant research results. Secure file sharing could be used to allow access to the EPR at any location, with changes automatically propagated back to the original database.

Security

The more computerised, networked and 'intelligent' our working environment becomes, the more vulnerable we become to error and malice. The security and reliability of present home/office machines and networks certainly leaves a lot to be desired and would not support the ambitious schemes discussed above.

One school of thought recommends secrecy and closure as a remedy for hackers and viruses. In this future the 'source code' or schematics for computer operating systems and applications will remain tightly guarded commercial secrets and this process of secrecy will be extended to the user's own hardware, which will contain tamper-proof monitoring devices inaccessible both technically and legally even to the owner of the computer (this is referred to as 'trusted hardware'). A favourable presentation of the idea from Microsoft is available at *http://www.microsoft.com/technet/archive/security/news/ngscb.mspx*.

Critics of this view charge that, far from empowering users, schemes for 'trusted computing' are in fact intended to safeguard the interests of large companies by preventing the unauthorised copying of media content and preventing leaks of embarrassing information by employees. According to these commentators, openness is the solution to both security problems and malfunctioning software. Only by having the full source code available for all to inspect can one be truly confident that a piece of software contains no errors likely to lead to failure or a breach of security. The Cambridge computer scientist Ross Anderson provides a critical analysis of the issues around trusted computing at *http://www.cl.cam.ac.uk/~rja14/tcpa-faq.html.*

This tension between open and closed, transparent and opaque will play itself out in many fields, some quite remote from computing, and may become one of the defining political issues of this century.

Human issues

Loneliness and dehumanisation

A future of autonomous intelligent software, of interaction by email and videoconferencing may be convenient but it may also erode the social supports available to the most vulnerable in our society, including those with a mental illness. What would be more worrying still would be the uncritical adoption, for resource reasons, of depersonalising technologies by mental health services as a substitute for, instead of an adjunct to, face-to-face contact.

Intrusion and the loss of solitude

Paradoxically, solitude can be hard to achieve in a world of depersonalised communication. Improvements in communication create a sort of connectivity arms race, in which we expect others to be instantly available to us while simultaneously resenting their demands on our own time.

The motto of the Royal College of Psychiatrists is 'Let wisdom guide'. True wisdom, however, is born of reflection, which in turn requires a quiet personal space. Such a space, an 'asylum' in the true sense, may be a rare commodity, for both patients and their doctors, in the years to come.

Threats to status

In other industries, the introduction of new, productivity-enhancing technologies is often associated with a reduction in the status of those working in that industry. As examples of this, consider the transformation of independent artisans into factory workers in 19th-century Britain or the changes in the UK printing industry in the early 1980s.

Similarly, technological developments such as videoconferencing and electronic patient records could lead to greater psychiatric 'productivity' at the expense of professional autonomy and work satisfaction. It might be a little far-fetched to imagine out-patient services being provided remotely from call centres but such 'outsourcing' and 'offshoring' have certainly affected the incomes of IT professionals in the past few years.

In addition, other, less expensive, professionals may be able to perform many of the tasks currently performed by psychiatrists if supported by IT systems and remote consultation.

The creation of 'expert patients' is also a goal being pursued by the current UK government as a way of managing costs and encouraging self-help. Improvements in the quality of online information, perhaps with the development of the semantic web, could support this trend, further eroding the professional role.

It might be, then, that the necessary corollary of the empowerment of patients and colleagues is the relative disempowerment of psychiatrists. If this process means more and better mental health care, then the psychiatric profession, in opposing it, will be in the same uncomfortable place once occupied by the Luddites or the striking print workers of Wapping.

The Panopticon

It will not have escaped notice that many of the technologies discussed above have immense potential for invading privacy. RFID tags could be used to track people as well as pets, financial records and closed-circuit television coverage could be scanned by neural networks or pattern-recognition engines for evidence of 'suspicious' behaviour and 'trusted' wearable computers running specialised remembrance agents could be a powerful tool of surveillance of both the wearer and others – a kind of supercharged electronic tag. The British author Charles Stross refers to this kind of massive automated surveillance as the 'Panopticon Singularity' and believes that it may happen in the near future.

If history tells us anything, it is that groups who are perceived as outsiders will be the first (though not the last) to be made subject to this kind of intrusive monitoring. Thus, we can expect the homeless, the mentally ill and asylum seekers to be among the 'early adopters' of this technology.

As psychiatrists we are in a position to oppose the current zeitgeist, this obsessional search for what Mason called 'safe certainty'. by calmly pointing out that, in fleeing the largely imaginary risks posed by the outsider, we may be embracing the far greater risks inherent in a surveillance state.

Further reading

Baer, L., Cukor, P., Jenike, M. A., *et al* (1995) Pilot studies of telemedicine for patients with obsessive–compulsive disorder. *American Journal of Psychiatry*, **152**, 1383–1385.

McClelland, I., Adamson, K. & Black, N. D. (1995) Information issues in telemedicine systems. *Journal of Telemedicine and Telecare*, **1**, 7–12.

Roine, R., Ohinmaa, A. & Hailey, D. (2001) Assessing telemedicine: a systematic review of the literature. *Canadian Medical Association Journal*, **165**, 765–771.

Yellowlees, P. (1997) Successful development of telemedicine systems – seven core principles. *Journal of Telemedicine and Telecare*, **3**, 215–222.

Yellowlees, P. (1997) The use of telemedicine to perform psychiatric assessments under the Mental Health Act. *Journal of Telemedicine and Telecare*, **3**, 224–226.

Index

Compiled by Caroline Sheard